CW01367577

KIDS, FAMILIES AND CHAOS

LIVING WITH ATTENTION DEFICIT DISORDER

By the same author

Stress Management: Teachers' Notes

Stress Management: A Compendium Of Techniques

Young People With Asthma: A Package Of Three Books
- . Beating Asthma: A Winner's Guide For Parents
- . Asthma - How To Become A Winner: A Student's Guide
- . Students With Asthma: How Schools Can Help

A Guide For Relaxation And Inner Mental Training
    (Co-authors - Elisabeth Solin & Lars Gunnar Solin)

Attention Deficit Disorder (Booklet)

Medication For Attention Deficit Disorder (Booklet)

Tourette Syndrome (Booklet)

KIDS, FAMILIES AND CHAOS

LIVING WITH ATTENTION DEFICIT DISORDER

Dr Harry Nash

ED·MED
PUBLISHERS

Australia

KIDS, FAMILIES AND CHAOS
LIVING WITH ATTENTION DEFICIT DISORDER

First published in Australia in 1994 by
Ed•Med Publishers
P.O. Box 303, Torrensville, South Australia, Australia   5031

© 1994 Harry Nash

Reprinted 1994

All rights reserved. No part of this publication may be reproduced, stored in a retrieval system, or transmitted, in any form or by any means, electronic, mechanical, photocopying, recording or otherwise without the prior permission of the publisher in writing.

Copies of this book may be ordered from the publisher.

Nash, Harry.
Kids, Families And Chaos
Living With Attention Deficit Disorder

ISBN   0 646 16978 5

Designed and illustrated by Jeff Rainsford and Harry Nash

Printed in Australia by Sports Guide Publications, Adelaide

To Rita, Toby and Josh
and in loving memory of
John and Sonia

SPECIAL ACKNOWLEDGEMENTS

The late Dr Gordon Serfontein was a great pioneer in the field of Attention Deficit Disorder. He brought this condition to the notice of Australians through his book *The Hidden Handicap*. His vision was to establish innovative centres for the assessment and management of children with this disability. He succeeded, in spite of immense opposition from many quarters. Gordon altered the lives of thousands of distressed children and families and they will surely be eternally indebted to him. Gordon inspired and encouraged me to set up practice in this field. I will be forever grateful to him. He died in his prime and before he could carry out even greater work. His book, *ADD in Adults*, was published after his death and this contribution will greatly benefit those adults who suffer from this significant disability.

Professor Garry Kneebone, a fine paediatrician and human being, has been of enormous help and support over many years. His understanding, empathy and patience have made it possible for me to continue in my work. I will always value his friendship.

ACKNOWLEDGEMENTS

I value greatly the continuing support of my medical colleagues, Ian Buttfield, Paul Duffy and Christopher Green. I thank Rosemary Deadman, Maria Grant, Max McQuillan, Rita Nash, Di Peake, Edith Pringle, Ros Phillips, Lyz Reynolds, Susan Secombe and Peter Webb for their invaluable suggestions and advice about the text. I appreciate the work of Jeff Rainsford, a respected friend and colleague, who designed and illustrated this book.

CONTENTS

Acknowledgements

Foreword

Introduction

Chapters

1	Types Of Attention Deficit Disorder	1
2	Behaviour And Development	11
3	About Attention Deficit Disorder	19
4	Temperament Of Children With Attention Deficit Disorder	29
5	The Behaviours Of Children With Attention Deficit Disorder	37
6	Different Situations - Different Behaviours	47
7	Conditions Related To Attention Deficit Disorder	53
8	Living With Attention Deficit Disorder	63
9	Families Of Children With Attention Deficit Disorder	69
10	Assessment Of Children With Attention Deficit Disorder	81
11	General Aspects Of Management	89
12	Medical Management	95
13	Psychological Management	103
14	Educational Strategies	115
15	The Future Of Children With Attention Deficit Disorder	127
16	Facts and Fallacies about Attention Deficit Disorder	135
17	Future Directions	143

Appendices 149

1 Specific Behavioural Aspects Of ADD 151
2 Assessment - Issues For Parents 157
3 Assessment - Teacher Issues 163
4 Benefits Of Medication 167
5 Some Specific Psychological Strategies 169
6 Skills Development 179
7 Varying Learning Strategies 183

References 187

FOREWORD

Attention Deficit Disorder (ADD) is a developmental disorder of behavioural inhibition which results in a pattern of symptoms in the areas of poor sustained attention and concentration, limited impulse control, and excessive activity level or hyperactivity. However, over time, other symptoms or deficits will emerge that are secondary to the core impairment in behavioural inhibition and which will greatly impact upon the person's ability to meet the many daily demands of family life, peer, school and employment settings.

These impairments will adversely affect: (1) the ability to organise behaviour over time so as to create difficulties in meeting future deadlines and commitments; (2) judging the passage of time normally and in using it to prepare for upcoming events; (3) reflecting upon both hindsight and forethought before determining the best course of action in a situation; (4) inhibiting initial emotional reactions to situations while evaluating the facts at hand (which I call separating facts from feelings); and (5) relying upon one's inner voice or language to help guide and control behaviour.

All of these five mental processes are essential to the development of self-control and serve to organise and direct behaviour toward future events. In doing so, they help the individual to maximise his or her future rewards and accomplishments while freeing the person up from excessive control by things happening in the immediate situation.

In short, what begins as a central problem with inhibiting behaviour in the child with ADD progresses to a developmental disorder in self-control that ultimately handicaps the individual's ability to direct behaviour toward the future so as to be effective in attaining future goals and rewards. The individual so disabled is left being more controlled by momentary circumstances, working mainly to maximise immediate gratification, unable to inhibit emotional reactions to events and people, and limited in the capacity for self-control or self-discipline.

That society would come to view the child with ADD as being immature, lazy, undisciplined, and even immoral, based on these patterns of social behaviour should not be surprising. What society does not recognise, however, is the underlying biological and often hereditary nature to this problem and the compassion for those with ADD which such a view would elicit.

But, gratefully, times are changing. Society is increasingly being educated about ADD and how it impacts upon the daily lives of several hundred thousand to one million children and adults in Australia who suffer from ADD. And become educated about ADD we must because those with the disorder constitute a large minority of the population that struggles and fails at school, that terminates schooling prematurely, that turns to antisocial behaviour and delinquency as well as early experimentation with illegal substances, that fails to sustain long-term relationships, and that underachieves at school and in the workplace.

The present book for parents makes a commendable contribution to this education of society. It provides an accurate, up-to-date body of information for parents and teachers on the nature of ADD in children and the things which may cause it. Equally as important, it directs parents and teachers in ways that they can use to help reduce the problems that children with ADD experience and to increase the success that these children will have in the family, in school, with peers, and in the larger community. It steers clear of the current closet of bogus remedies, shams, fads, and other unproven or disproven treatments despite the widespread popularity for some, such as the notion that eliminating sugar from the child's diet helps treat ADD. Yet it provides the essential details of effective home and school management methods for use with ADD children and also gives us a no-nonsense account of how useful certain medications may be for many children with this disorder.

I congratulate Dr Harry Nash on his witty style, entertaining prose, imaginative graphics and sensible information to be found in this wonderful book for families with ADD children. I am honoured to be asked to contribute in some small way to his laudable efforts to educate others on behalf of children with ADD and to provide reasonable and effective advice to the families who must raise such children in the face of a society that erroneously doubts its existence.

But prevail we must.

Russell A. Barkley, Ph.D.
Director of Psychology
Professor of Psychiatry and Neurology
University of Massachusetts Medical Centre
Worcester, Massachusetts   U.S.A.

INTRODUCTION

There has been considerable media coverage about Attention Deficit Disorder (ADD) recently. Hardly a week goes by without some reference to ADD in newspapers, magazines, radio or television. Some people wonder if this 'new wave epidemic' is a passing fad. Others may consider that the label can be applied to all children who experience any type of behaviour or learning problem.

In fact, ADD is not a new epidemic. It has affected people for centuries. This very common disability has only recently come to the notice of the public, and more of us are recognising that it can be a great problem for many children, their families and teachers.

Children with ADD are 'different'. The condition makes it more difficult for them to pay attention and to control their behaviour, things which other children can do easily, naturally and with little effort. Their disability is often complicated by the negative responses from other people. Their parents, brothers and sisters, teachers and school mates find it difficult to understand how they 'tick', how best to help them, and how to manage their own reactions and frustrations.

These young people have a physiological problem involving a part of the brain which does not operate in an efficient way. This results in poor self-control and a range of difficulties that may show up as various obstacles to learning and in controlling behaviour. They are at a disadvantage and constantly struggle in an attempt to overcome this lack of self-control.

These children often suffer great obstacles in their ability to cope in a range of areas. ADD can result in inappropriate learning, behaviour and socialisation styles. Over and above all of this, their poor self esteem, stress reactions and poor school progress may contribute to a significant handicap. Many of them experience difficulties in relating to their families and peers.

These children are often a mystery and an enigma to the people around them. They may be labelled as being 'lazy', 'rude', 'irresponsible', 'inconsiderate', 'moody', 'disruptive', or 'dumb'. They are often easily frustrated and they are frustrating to others. They find it difficult to fit in socially. These young people, however, are not 'problem children', but rather 'children who have a problem'.

The word 'chaos' in the title of this book has been deliberately chosen. Children with ADD often find themselves in crisis and in a predicament of confusion and disorganisation. The same is true of their families, teachers and others who try their best to assist them. They are often at their wit's end in trying to find the key to guide these children to achieve their potential.

Many parents and teachers become confused because the usual strategies that work for other children simply do not work for those with ADD. They are often frustrated because of their failed efforts to help these children who suffer from a puzzling and often a significant disability.

Many of these children experience repeated failure in many areas of their lives. If their disability is not identified and managed properly in their early years, there is a possibility that many of them and their families are likely to tread down a path of continuing stress and major setbacks for many years.

ADD is also a very significant public health issue, since it has ramifications not only for affected children and their families, but also the society in which they live. It is a condition which is potentially destructive to the well-being and self-esteem of these children. If left untreated, it may contribute to a range of major learning difficulties and emotional problems. It may also contribute to antisocial behaviour. This raises important questions about the rehabilitation of distressed people and the costs of providing these services in the community. Yet, ADD is a treatable condition and these complications can often be prevented.

The aim of this book is to help people understand and recognise the difficulties experienced by children with ADD. The information presented in this book is based on the most recent practical research. Once the condition is properly understood and managed, the future of these children and their families is very likely to be greatly improved. Early and accurate assessment and treatment are the important keys for a more positive outcome. The negative spiral of poor self-esteem, failure and damaged relationships may be prevented with early intervention.

For ease of expression, the terms 'he', 'his' and 'him' will be used throughout the text to describe children with ADD. More boys than girls are recognised as suffering from this condition.

I never think of the future. It comes soon enough   Albert Einstein

As the occasion, so the behaviour   Cervantes *Don Quixote*

Soon learnt, soon forgotten   Proverb

I had nothing to offer anybody except my own confusion
                                    Jack Kerouac *On the Road*

This form of therapy (the use of stimulant medication) is so well proven it is no longer worth debating this point. Some people still believe the world is flat, but that's not our problem
                                    Dr Christopher Green

CHAPTER 1

TYPES OF ATTENTION DEFICIT DISORDER

> **Summary**
>
> There are two types of ADD -
>
> Attention Deficit Disorder with Hyperactivity or ADD(+H),
> and
> Attention Deficit Disorder without hyperactivity or ADD(-H).
>
> The two scenarios describe the main features of each type of ADD.

Chapter 1: Types of Attention Deficit Disorder

Two Types Of Attention Deficit Disorder

There are two main types of ADD. One is named **Attention Deficit Disorder with Hyperactivity**. The other type is known as **Attention Deficit Disorder without hyperactivity**. They differ from each other in several ways but are similar in other respects.

Children who suffer from **Attention Deficit with Hyperactivity**, or **ADD(+H)**, have difficulties in focusing and sustaining their attention, and they also have problems in controlling their muscle activity (often called 'hyperactivity') and in regulating behaviour (usually called 'impulsiveness'). These children are often easily identified because they are restless and frequently create difficulties for others as a result of their disruptiveness and 'difficult' temperament. They have been called 'Fidgety Phil', 'Fast Freddy' or 'Speedy Gonzales'. Although many children with ADD(+H) outgrow their hyperactivity with increasing maturity of their nervous system, a significant number continue to experience difficulties in paying attention and various other aspects of their ADD.

The main difficulties faced by children with **Attention Deficit Disorder without hyperactivity** or **ADD(-H)** are the result of poor selective and poor sustained attention. They have few, if any, problems in controlling their behaviour and they are not hyperactive. These children, unfortunately, often go unrecognised because they are usually quiet and do not create problems for others. They are often labelled as 'daydreamers'. Their difficulties in focusing and sustaining attention frequently result in poor academic achievement.

Two Scenarios

The following stories are typical of two children. They are a composite of the information that parents often bring to the attention of doctors, psychologists and counsellors. It is hoped that these descriptions will help people become aware of, and more familiar with, the two main types of ADD. Each scenario will be followed by key points which will be expanded in later chapters.

Chapter 1: Types of Attention Deficit Disorder

Scenario 1
Attention Deficit Disorder With Hyperactivity
Or ADD(+H)

Dean's parents have been exasperated by their son's difficult behaviour since birth. Even when his mother was pregnant, he was very active in the womb and his constant kicking and movement caused a great deal of discomfort for her. As a baby he was a very fussy feeder and did not need very much sleep. He was an irritable and demanding baby and he cried constantly. His parents were told that he was suffering from colic.

When he was a toddler his parents were informed that his behaviour was normal - 'the terrible twos' - and that he would grow out of it. But he continued to be very difficult. Various people such as friends, neighbours and other family members offered advice that made Dean's parents feel awful - 'don't worry'; 'give him more love and attention'; 'he needs a good thrashing'; 'see a counsellor'; 'change his diet and take out artificial colourings'; 'try time out'; 'do a parenting course'; 'he's just an active boy'; 'he'll grow out of it'; 'put him on tranquillisers'. They tried many of these suggestions, but none of them were effective.

They did wait, but he did not grow out of it. The terrible twos became the terrible threes and fours and fives. His speech and language seemed a little immature, and he appeared clumsy at times. Sometimes he was a real pleasure to be with and could do things quite easily. On other days, however, his behaviour was very irritating and difficult to manage, and he could not do the simplest of tasks, even though he had done them the previous day without any difficulties. The old saying 'when he is good he's very, very good .... and when he is bad he is horrid' certainly applied to Dean.

Dean was a human dynamo. He woke very early and went at a hundred miles an hour all day. Nothing satisfied him, even though his parents gave him all the love and attention they could offer. They tried to satisfy his needs, but he just demanded more and more attention. He became easily bored with things that did not interest him, and both his parents noticed that he was more restless and frustrated at these times.

Chapter 1: Types of Attention Deficit Disorder

He threw temper tantrums whenever his mother asked him to carry out simple requests such as getting dressed or eating meals at the dinner table. Some of the things he did were very dangerous. He played with scissors and knives, and on several occasions he tried to cut through electrical cords connected to the power supply. He had little concept of danger and often climbed trees and ladders to get on to the roof of the house.

He continued his perilous behaviours in spite of repeated explanations about the dangers of his actions. Shopping at the supermarket was nerve racking as he ran amok in an uncontrolled manner, creating havoc for his mother, other shoppers and the staff. This frequently happened when he didn't get his own way, for example when he wanted a piece of candy and his mother refused to comply with his demands.

Dean had trouble paying attention and he did not seem to listen. His attention often shifted from one thing to another, usually to those things that were more interesting than the boring or uninteresting tasks he was asked to carry out. He forgot almost immediately what was requested of him, especially when he was already doing something enjoyable such as watching television.

There were some things that did not trouble him. He played with his building equipment happily and he was delightful when he played on his own or with one other friend. He was usually cooperative with his father and when he received individual attention.

When Dean was four years old, he started at kindergarten. His behaviour was rather aggressive at times and his teacher noticed that his attention wandered. He repeatedly did silly things without thinking about them first, and his behaviour often interfered with what the other children were doing. After some time they began to avoid Dean because of his loudness and aggressive outbursts. They sometimes retaliated and Dean could not understand why he was unpopular.

Dean's parents took him to a number of experts who reassured them that he was a normal boy and that there was nothing to worry about. They included the general practitioner, paediatricians, psychologists and different advisers and counsellors.

Chapter 1: Types of Attention Deficit Disorder

His parents felt that there was something wrong, but no one seemed to listen to their concerns nor suggest ways to help in managing Dean's difficult behaviour. They tried everything the books recommended, but nothing really worked for any length of time.

Their patience became exhausted and they could not agree on how best to handle Dean. They often blamed one another out of sheer exasperation and frustration. Dean's irritating, troublesome and aggressive behaviour continued to be a major problem. His parents did not know what else to do.

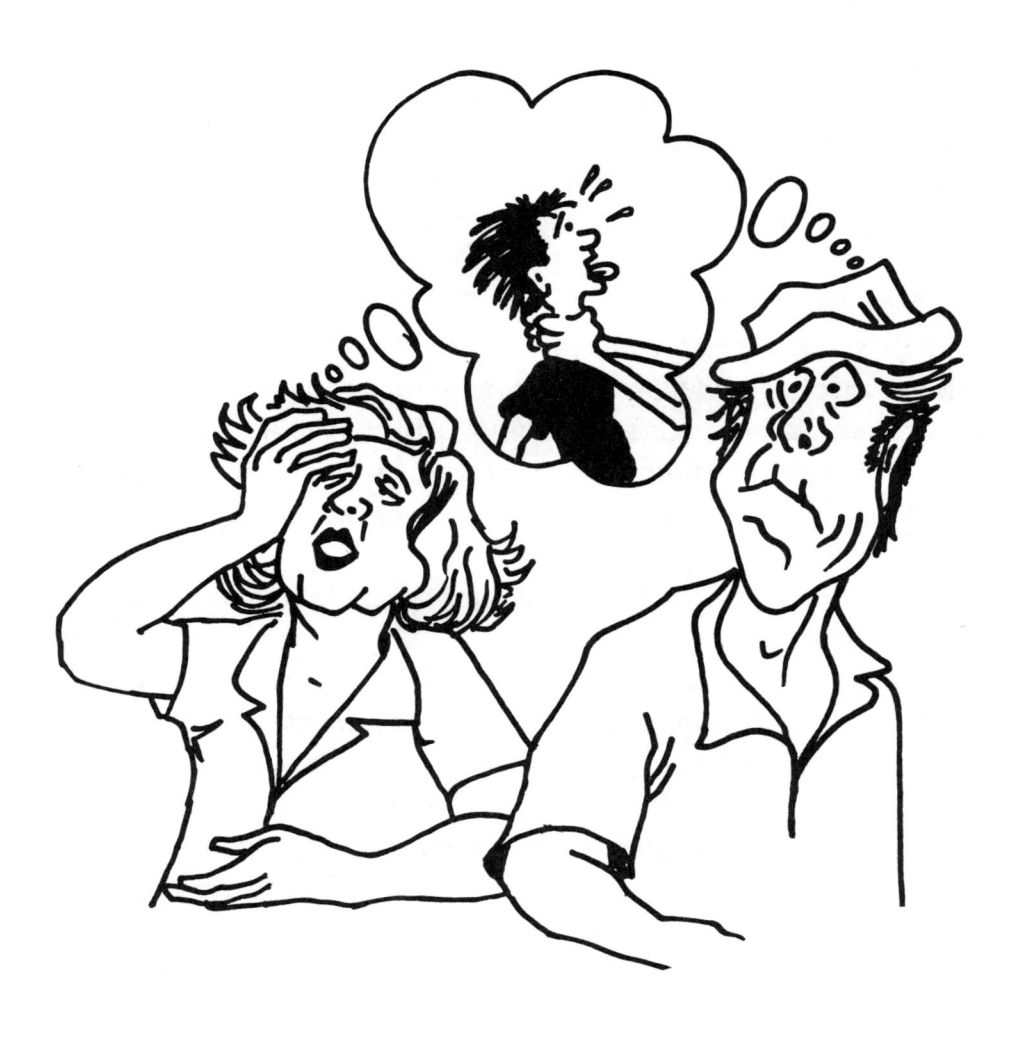

Chapter 1: Types of Attention Deficit Disorder

Dean started school and he settled in quite well. However, after several weeks his behaviour became increasingly annoying to the other students. Although he wanted to make friends with the other students, he could not develop any friendships because the other children didn't like the things he did to them.

He was disruptive in the classroom and he was easily distracted. He became easily frustrated at the slightest provocation, and his short fuse frequently led to aggressive outbursts toward anyone who asked him to cooperate.

He constantly got into trouble in the classroom and playground. He became the class clown and he repeatedly received 'time out' for his rather dangerous, impulsive and antisocial behaviour. He was asked to see the principal regularly and was given frequent detentions. Dean was the regular discussion topic of teachers in the staff room at lunchtime. He developed the reputation of being a nuisance to teachers and students and Dean was labelled as a troublemaker and a poor learner. These labels stuck !

Whenever there was any trouble at school, Dean was automatically blamed. His teachers had difficulties in keeping him on task and encouraging him to complete his schoolwork. The other students soon realised that they could get Dean into trouble easily, and they often 'baited' him. He was suspended on several occasions. No method of discipline was effective, and certainly the school discipline policy was of little value when applied to Dean.

His parents knew that Dean had great capabilities and potential. He had good days and he was absolutely brilliant when using the computer. He was also often a loving and caring child. But everything he did, or didn't do, caused pain and suffering to his parents and himself. And they could see that he was a very unhappy and unpopular child with very poor confidence and self-esteem.

His parents became increasingly demanding and they tried to force Dean to do things in an attempt to help him become better organised and to cooperate and carry out their requests. These 'tough' tactics only made matters worse. Dean became more defiant and aggressive. They ran out of ideas and options and considered themselves failures as parents. The climate at home became increasingly tense, hostile and unhappy.

Chapter 1: Types of Attention Deficit Disorder

Dean's parents thought seriously about his future and they repeatedly asked themselves:

'Will he ever become a capable learner ?'
'How can we help him feel better about himself ?'
'How can he learn to keep out of trouble ?'
'Will he become a social misfit ?'
'How can we help him to make friends ?'
'Will he be able to find a reasonable job ?'

Key Points In Scenario 1

- Dean's problems with temperament and behaviour were evident from a very early age.
- It was difficult to keep him satisfied.
- He had difficulties in controlling his behaviour and in focusing his attention on relevant tasks and activities. Dean's behaviour was unpredictable and often seemed to be outside his control.
- His performance and effort were erratic or inconsistent. He carried out some activities very well but had great difficulties with others.
- He was better able to pay attention and control his behaviour in some situations, but found it more difficult to be in control in others. Dean's self-control was better when there were few demands placed on him and when he received individual attention. He had difficulties when given instructions, particularly when there were more interesting things for him to do.
- Many of the methods tried by his parents and teachers were either only partially helpful or totally unsuccessful.
- The diagnosis of ADD was not considered in Dean's early years of life.
- Dean's difficulties in controlling attention and behaviour led to a variety of problems. He was in constant trouble at school and had difficulty in keeping friends. He fell behind in his schoolwork, even though it was obvious that he was quite intelligent. His self-esteem deteriorated and he was very unhappy.
- The family was put under considerable stress. They had great fears for his future in terms of his school progress, career options, social relationships and emotional well-being.

Chapter 1: Types of Attention Deficit Disorder

Scenario 2 :

Attention Deficit Disorder Without Hyperactivity Or ADD(-H)

Kate was a rather quiet and shy girl. She was cooperative and always a delight to be with. As a young girl Kate was a 'dreamer'. Her parents thought that she was deep in thought. When they asked her to do things around the house, Kate did not seem to listen to their requests and she seemed rather forgetful. But they did not think that this was a great problem, even though they needed to get her attention and repeat instructions several times before she carried them out. She liked playing on her own, particularly when other people came to visit.

At school Kate was also rather quiet. She had one or two close friends and they enjoyed her company. Her teachers found Kate to be a very pleasant student. However, by grade 4 it became obvious that she was falling behind in her schoolwork. Her teachers noticed that Kate was easily distracted by things happening in the classroom. She found it difficult to focus on tasks that required her to pay attention for long periods. She was rather disorganised and lost track of her pencils, books and other materials needed to carry out various tasks and activities in the classroom.

Kate also lost track of the teacher's instructions and sometimes asked the teacher to repeat them. She found it difficult to get started on her work and often did not get it finished. Her writing was untidy and she made silly mistakes in her work, particularly in arithmetic calculations and spelling.

Kate didn't seem to listen and her teachers thought that she was preoccupied and in a world of her own. They needed to supervise her work closely so that she would stay on task.

All her school reports had variations on the same theme: 'Kate is a cooperative member of the class. Capable of doing much better. Fails to finish assigned tasks. Needs to learn to concentrate and organise herself'.

Chapter 1: Types of Attention Deficit Disorder

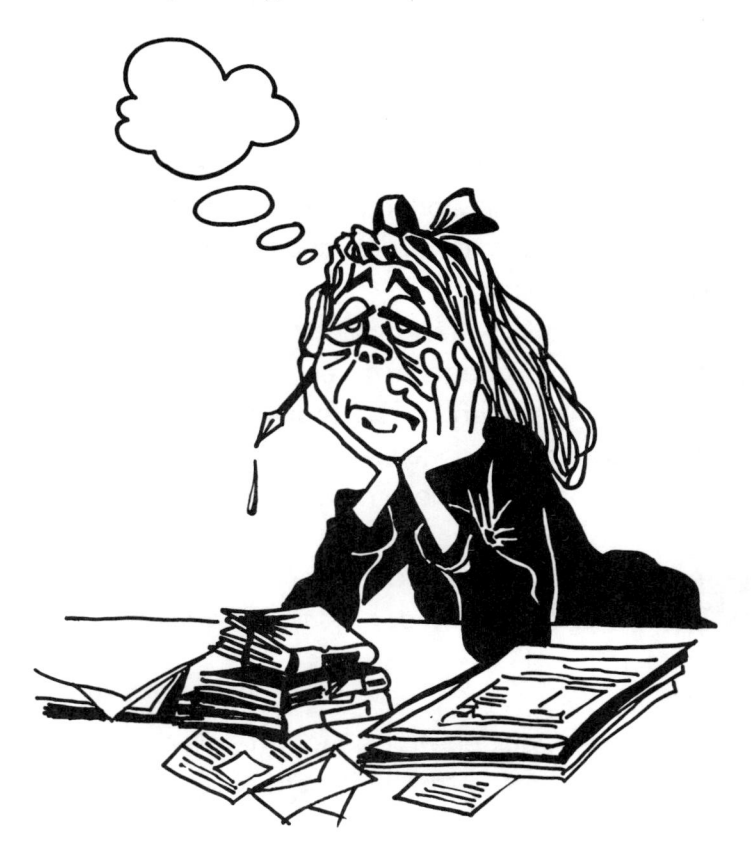

Her school performance and progress became a great concern for her parents and teachers. Kate's confidence and self-esteem soon deteriorated, especially when she recognised that she was not doing as well as the other students in the class. She often spent hours on school assignments and trying to learn her maths tables and spelling. This was difficult work for her and also for her parents who spent a great deal of time trying to help her. They all became very frustrated when, in spite of all the time and effort devoted to her work, by the next day Kate had forgotten most of what she had learned the night before.

Kate was asked to repeat a grade because of her poor progress. Everyone knew she was an intelligent girl because there were days when she performed very well in many aspects of her work. On other days she achieved very little.

Her parents did not know how to help. Kate was assessed by several different specialists who told the family that she was a slow learner and that she needed to put more effort into her work.

Chapter 1: Types of Attention Deficit Disorder

Key Points In Scenario 2

- There were few, if any, clues to indicate that Kate was experiencing difficulties until long after she started school. Her quiet and shy nature and the early warning signs of forgetfulness and daydreaming were not considered to be problems.
- Kate's difficulties in paying attention and staying on task became more obvious when schoolwork began to overwhelm her. Her problems in focusing and sustaining attention resulted in academic underachievement.
- Her effort and work performance were inconsistent. Sometimes she performed well, whereas at other times she did poorly.
- Her self-esteem gradually deteriorated.
- Kate's parents and teachers found it difficult to come up with strategies to help her. Family stress increased as a result of the parents' impotence to assist her.

These two scenarios set the scene for a more detailed discussion about ADD. They have highlighted some of the various problems experienced by these children, their families and teachers. A more thorough description about ADD will be presented after the important subject of normal development and behaviour is considered in the next chapter.

CHAPTER 2

BEHAVIOUR AND DEVELOPMENT

> **Summary**
>
> Brain development depends on many factors.
>
> The various parts of the brain can carry out their intended functions only when the electrical/chemical system operates in a mature way.
>
> Delay in maturation may create problems in the way the various parts of the brain operate.
>
> ADD is the result of delayed maturation of a part of the brain.

Chapter 2: Behaviour And Development

About Development

Development is a process of maturation which depends on many different and connected factors. Some of these include heredity, events during pregnancy and birth, hormones, nutrition, culture and family background, physical health, relationships with parents, as well as early experiences with various people and events. All these factors shape how we grow and mature. They are important in the development of our intelligence, language, emotions, temperament and personality, muscle coordination, relationships with others and many other activities and functions.

When brain development goes according to plan, and the various parts of the brain connect with one another, the nerve cells or neurons can work properly in an organised and efficient way. Electrical signals are sent along these neurons and these impulses allow certain chemical messengers, or neurotransmitters, to pass from one cell to the next in an orderly fashion. This electrical/chemical system sends messages to relevant parts of the brain so that they can carry out their intended functions. When this occurs in the appropriate way, the relevant action or behaviour is produced.

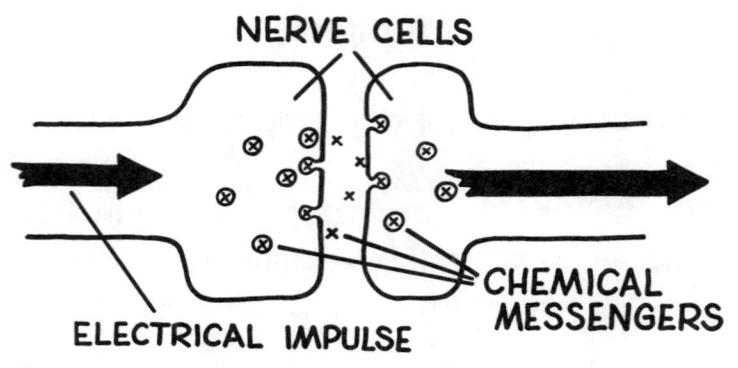

NERVE CELLS

ELECTRICAL IMPULSE — **CHEMICAL MESSENGERS**

Our brain serves many different purposes, but it can only operate properly when the electrical/chemical system works in an efficient and effective manner. Different areas of the brain and their connections are involved in carrying out many different, varied and often complicated functions. These include vision, thinking, speech and language, hearing and listening, feeling emotions, and moving the various parts of our body. These functions can only be carried out successfully if the connected and special areas of the brain are 'switched on' and ready to perform their intended work.

Chapter 2: Behaviour And Development

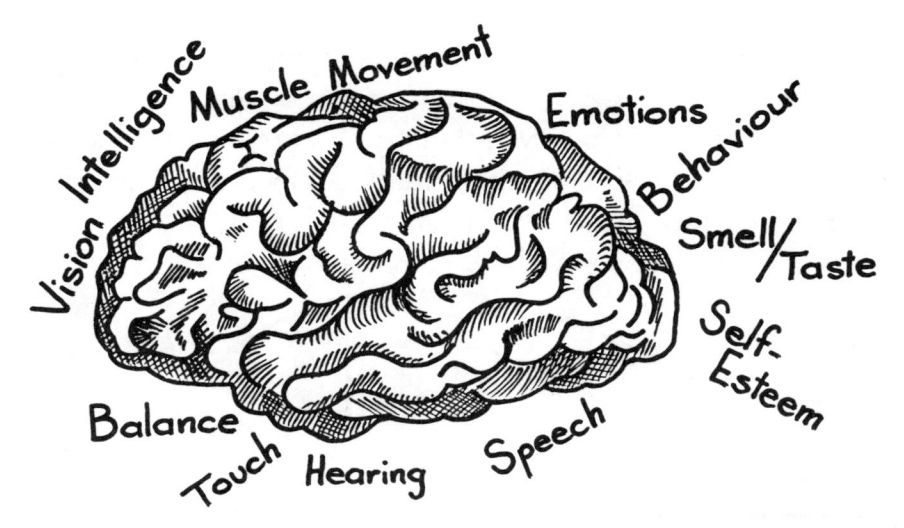

[Illustration of a brain labelled with: Vision, Intelligence, Muscle Movement, Emotions, Behaviour, Smell/Taste, Self-Esteem, Speech, Hearing, Touch, Balance]

In other words, various behaviours and skills can only be carried out if the particular areas of the brain involved have matured and developed properly. This enables the mature electrical and chemical equipment to work effectively.

If the system remains immature, then the involved area cannot work in the proper way and the desired behaviour cannot be carried out. This explains why babies and toddlers are unable to perform many of the activities and tasks that older children and adults are able to carry out automatically and with ease. Their brain's electrical/chemical system is simply not ready nor mature enough to perform the intended work of that particular area of the brain.

Control Of Behaviour

Behaviour is controlled or regulated by a feedback loop. One part of this loop involves an activation, stimulation or 'excitation' limb, which allows us to get started and ready to do various things. When this is operating properly we are able to choose and focus on the most suitable thing to do, start doing it, and continue until it is finished. It 'gets us moving', in a way similar to the accelerator speeding up a car.

There is another important part of the loop, and this allows us to check what we are doing and slow down if necessary, so that we can revise our tactics and change course when appropriate. This is the 'inhibitory' limb of the loop, and it works in a way similar to the brakes of a car, enabling it to slow down or stop. However, the nerve equipment controlling this part of behaviour control has to be mature and operating properly so that it may work in an efficient way. (It is the immaturity in the inhibitory limb of the feedback loop which is considered to be a fundamental problem for children with ADD).

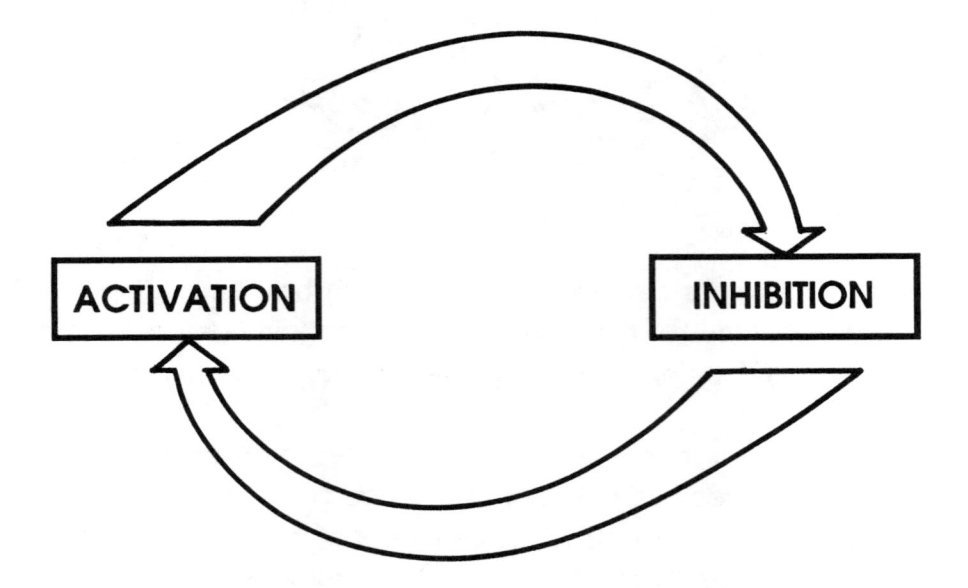

```
ACTIVATION  ⇄  INHIBITION
```

This feedback loop, the constant exchange of information between stimulation and inhibition, allows us to make rapid and almost automatic decisions about our behaviour. It allows us to determine what needs to be done from moment to moment so that we can adjust our behaviour accordingly.

The feedback loop works for most of us in an almost unconscious way. We often don't need to think about things that need to be done. We simply carry them out because they are second nature to us, a habit, just as we know when to use the accelerator and brakes when driving a car.

Elements Of Behaviour

Some important components of behaviour need to be emphasised. Most of us take these for granted because they are automatic and come very naturally and easily to us. These critical elements are:

Chapter 2: Behaviour And Development

- **Selective attention** - choosing the most relevant activity to focus on
- **Sustained attention** - continuing to focus on this activity over time
- **Rejecting or blocking out distractions** or unnecessary stimuli
- **Understanding and interpreting** relevant information
- **Setting goals** - deciding where we want to go
- **Planning and organising** - working out the necessary steps required to achieve these goals
- **Initiation** - starting off the necessary task or activity
- **Checking, modifying and regulating** activities and behaviour
- **Persistence of effort**
- **Completion** - finishing the task and arriving at the intended goal

These elements or components of behaviour are governed by the feedback loop described above. They are very important and allow us to be in control of the many activities, tasks and behaviours in which we are likely to be involved.

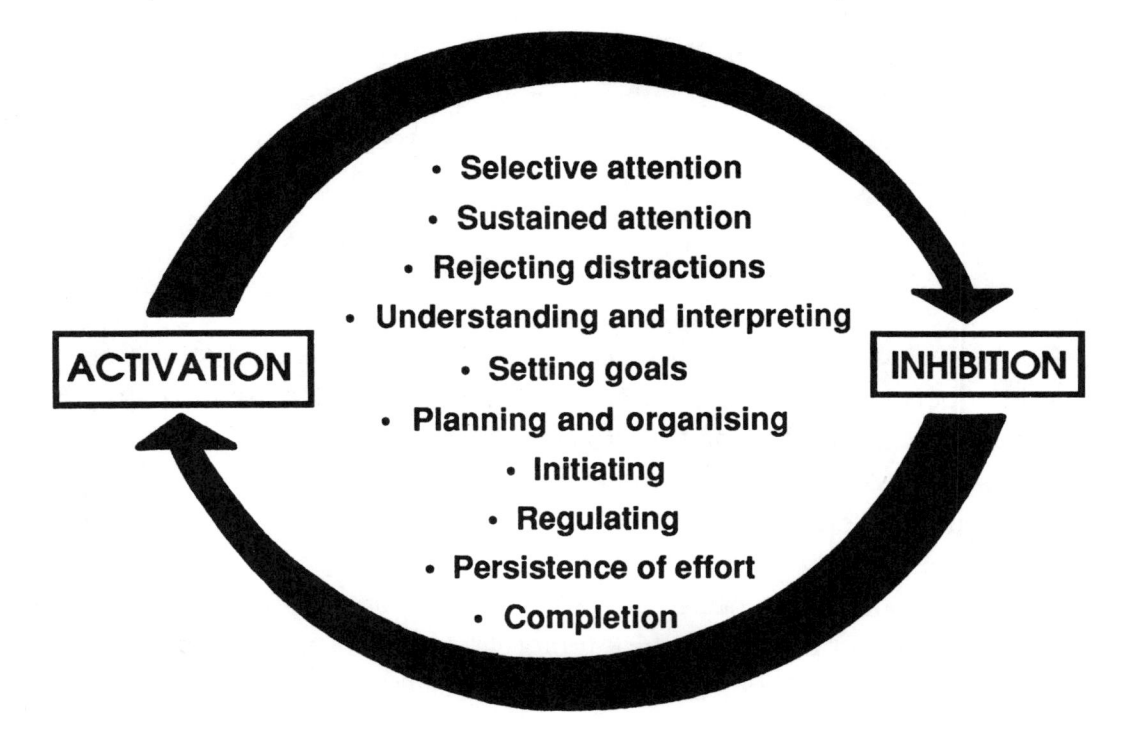

ACTIVATION ⇄ **INHIBITION**

- Selective attention
- Sustained attention
- Rejecting distractions
- Understanding and interpreting
- Setting goals
- Planning and organising
- Initiating
- Regulating
- Persistence of effort
- Completion

Chapter 2: Behaviour And Development

When these components of behaviour work for us in positive ways we are able to control and regulate most behaviours including a variety of: activities, tasks and chores; specific skills and abilities; emotions and moods; muscle activity and coordination; and social behaviour.

If the activation and inhibition functions of the feedback loop do not work in tandem, then major difficulties in various aspects of behaviour may result. This is what happens with many toddlers who have not yet developed the capacity to inhibit their behaviours. This is the reason why many of them are 'constantly on the go', 'always into everything', 'don't pay attention' and 'often in trouble'.

They cannot put on the brakes because the loop's inhibition limb has not yet developed properly, and because of this they cannot control their behaviour to the same extent as older children and adults. This inhibition function develops over time and, with maturity, it enables us to take increasing control over various aspects of our behaviour.

In many ways, the behaviour of children with ADD is similar to that observed in toddlers. The inhibition limb of their feedback loop is not as well developed as the activation limb. And it is this which produces many of their difficulties. They experience a range of problems as a result of their difficulty in regulating and controlling various aspects of their behaviour. These are likely to impinge on various people who must learn to cope with the 'uncontrolled' behaviour.

Temperament

Our behaviour is also influenced by our unique and individual temperament, style or personality. Some people are shy and timid, others are more outgoing and friendly, and still others tend to have a 'short fuse' and are irritable. These different styles affect the way we get on with other people and how we respond in various situations.

The temperaments of children with ADD are very different when compared to other children and this important factor will be discussed in Chapter 4: 'The Temperaments Of Children With Attention Deficit Disorder'.

Chapter 2: Behaviour And Development

Situations Can Influence Behaviour

Our behaviours are also influenced by the different types of situations in which we find ourselves. These situations usually include people, activities, and the various objects and other materials that surround us. Circumstances change as we move from one setting to another. We are likely to adjust our behaviour according to the situation at hand and the time of day. For example, we usually act quite differently with our friends at a party compared to the way we behave at home when alone watching television, studying in a class or carrying out some work in an office or factory.

Children with ADD frequently experience greater difficulties in some situations and not in others. This fact is important to appreciate because it may be critical in the management of these children. These important situational factors will be discussed in Chapter 6: 'Different Situations - Different Behaviours'.

CHAPTER 3

ABOUT ATTENTION DEFICIT DISORDER

> **Summary**
>
> ADD is common and is more frequently diagnosed in boys than in girls.
>
> Recent research suggests that the two types of ADD are different.
>
> A new model incorporates the important factors involved in children with ADD - their temperament, their poor behavioural control, and the situational variables that can influence them.

Chapter 3 : About Attention Deficit Disorder

Research Findings

The area of the brain involved in self-control and regulation of behaviour and attention operates in an immature way in children with ADD. As a result of this immaturity, the electrical/chemical system works in a less efficient way than it should. This results in the problems experienced by children with ADD.

Research shows that children with ADD have a physiological difficulty which affects this part of the brain which is located in the front portion of the brain. A special scanning method, known as positron emission tomography (PET), has demonstrated that there is a reduced blood flow and poor sugar metabolism, or decreased uptake of glucose, in this area of the brain.

Although there is a definite physiological problem in children with ADD, their difficulties in controlling their behaviour and attention are greatly influenced by different situations and environments. These situational factors include other people, activities and a range of different stimuli. This is a finding which is similar for people who suffer from other medical conditions such as migraine headaches, asthma, and diabetes, all of which may be either influenced in positive or adverse ways by what is happening around them or to them.

In the case of the child with ADD, such factors influence his self-control and the way he behaves and pays attention. Some situations enable him to improve or enhance his self-control, whereas others are more likely to create difficulties in his ability to regulate his behaviour.

A New Way Of Looking At Attention Deficit Disorder

The traditional way of defining ADD as the 'holy trinity' of poor concentration, hyperactivity and impulsiveness is becoming less useful. It was once thought that these were the fundamental symptoms in ADD. However, the most recent research shows that there is a more basic problem which affects the child with ADD. This involves difficulties with self-control and in the regulation of important elements of behaviour.

Chapter 3 : About Attention Deficit Disorder

His problems in regulating attention, both selective and sustained attention, are often interpreted by others as 'poor concentration'; his difficulty in controlling muscle activity is often called 'hyperactivity'; and the difficulty in regulating his general behaviour is often classified as 'impulsiveness'.

But such interpretations do not point to the basic problem encountered by the child with ADD. These terms do not take into account the difference between the two types of ADD, ADD with Hyperactivity or ADD(+H) and ADD without hyperactivity or ADD(-H).

The new way of looking at Attention Deficit Disorder is this:

ADD results from a developmental immaturity of that part of the brain which is involved in the self-control and regulation of behaviour in certain situations, especially those which involve rules, instructions or requests.

In other words he is likely to experience difficulties when it comes to starting and sustaining suitable behaviour in response to certain requests, instructions and tasks. This is especially difficult for him if there are other competing stimuli and more interesting things to do, or when the incentives or rewards for carrying out the task are not powerful enough. He has difficulties in inhibiting or blocking out certain behaviours when rewards are not given immediately, and if they are too weak or unimportant to him. In particular he is less likely to respond to those incentives or rewards which would influence most other children.

The following example may help illustrate these important points:

Tom needed to get ready so that his mother could get him to school on time. She asked him to get dressed and then pack his bag for school while he was watching his favourite early morning television program. He did not respond to her request. She became increasingly angry and frustrated because he did not carry out her instruction. She shouted and threatened him, in an attempt to gain his cooperation and get organised.

This episode may be explained in the following way. Tom's mother issued a request and the incentive was that he was to go to school. This was a rather weak incentive when compared to the more interesting and stimulating one of

Chapter 3 : About Attention Deficit Disorder

watching a television program. Her shouting was not a powerful consequence and it did not help the situation. (However, if she gave the instruction in a more positive and powerful way, or offered an incentive which was more important to him, it is more likely that he would have responded in a more suitable way).

A Model Of Attention Deficit Disorder

We can summarise the important factors involved in children with ADD by using the following model:

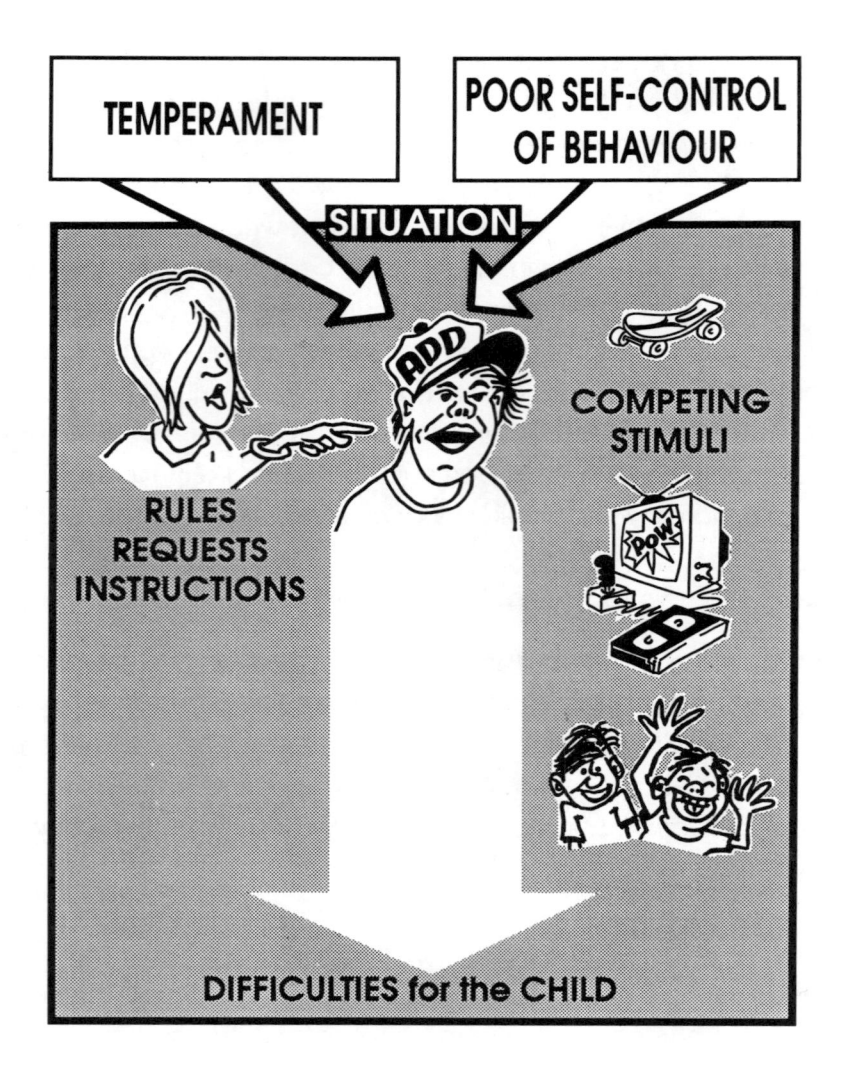

TEMPERAMENT

POOR SELF-CONTROL OF BEHAVIOUR

SITUATION

RULES REQUESTS INSTRUCTIONS

COMPETING STIMULI

DIFFICULTIES for the CHILD

Chapter 3 : About Attention Deficit Disorder

This model shows the important factors involved in ADD; that is, the interactions between:

- the temperament and behavioural aspects of the child with ADD
- the child in different situations
- requests and instructions given to the child on the one hand, and other competing stimuli in the environment or situation

These individual factors will be discussed in the following chapters.

Features Of Attention Deficit Disorder

The symptoms of ADD consist of a range of difficulties in which self-control is normally important. Therefore ADD may be seen as problems in: focusing and sustaining attention; initiating certain relevant tasks; modifying behaviour when necessary; planning and organising various activities; persistence of effort; and completion of tasks.

These will be discussed in more detail in Chapter 5: 'The Behaviours Of Children With Attention Deficit Disorder'.

The symptoms of ADD vary a great deal in the same child. Some of the factors that influence the condition include the time of day, the type of situation, the task or behaviour that needs to be carried out, as well as the people and other stimuli or distractions in the immediate situation.

This variation in behaviour is a very important matter, and it helps explain why some situations provide him with a much greater opportunity to control his behaviour. Another situation, on the other hand, may tax his problems with self-control and result in significant difficulties in self-control of behaviour and attention.

He is more vulnerable in several areas because he is 'machine driven' by an immature area of the brain. He has less control over his behaviour than other children. Yet, his intelligence and various other brain functions operate in a very normal way.

Chapter 3 : About Attention Deficit Disorder

This is a major disadvantage for him because he has the potential but can't use it in a consistent way. He often tries very hard to do the right thing, but he is let down repeatedly. He is likely to behave like a much younger child, and those methods that usually encourage and motivate positive behaviour and ability to pay attention in other children are less likely to work well for him.

ADD is a chronic or long lasting condition which starts in early childhood and is usually apparent before the age of 7 years. Other conditions such as severe intellectual disability, autism, major emotional stress or family upheaval, and hearing or visual impairment need to be excluded because these conditions sometimes result in a similar picture. Symptoms must be present for a minimum of 6 months before a diagnosis of ADD can be made with confidence.

Although some of the symptoms may improve as he gets older, the child with ADD is likely to experience difficulties into his teenage years and perhaps into adult life. Even when such improvement occurs, there are usually continuing differences between the child with ADD and other children in terms of control of behaviour and attention.

Cause Of Attention Deficit Disorder

Researchers have tried to discover the cause of ADD for many years. Their various theories and suggestions have included problems during pregnancy or birth, brain injury, infection of the brain, lead poisoning and other chemical sensitivities, sensitivity to certain foods and artificial colourings, poor parenting and many others. These theories have been shown to be generally incorrect.

Heredity has been shown to be the single most important cause of ADD. Quite often the child with ADD has a family member, perhaps one of his parents, who had ADD as a child or may even continue to experience some evidence of the condition as an adult. His brother or sister may also have ADD which may not be recognised. Interestingly, in sets of identical twins, if one twin has ADD then the other is very likely to be affected as well. The incidence of ADD is much higher in non-identical twins than in the general population. Such findings support the notion of ADD as an hereditary condition.

Chapter 3 : About Attention Deficit Disorder

Differences Between The Two Types Of ADD

It was once thought that the two types of ADD were variations of the same condition. Recent research suggests that ADD(+H) and ADD(-H) are probably different and distinct conditions. Further studies are needed to confirm this.

Children who have ADD(+H) are different from those with ADD(-H) in a number of ways:

- they differ in terms of their behaviour patterns and profiles
- their temperaments are quite different
- the areas of the brain involved are probably different. Research suggests that children with ADD(+H) have a functional problem in the front area of the brain, whereas the area involved in ADD(-H) is located further back in the brain
- there is probably a difference in the type of chemical messengers involved in each type of ADD. It is proposed that there is a reduced supply of dopamine in the affected brain cells in children with ADD(+H). In children with ADD(-H), there is less availability of a different chemical messenger, noradrenaline.

How Common Is Attention Deficit Disorder ?

ADD is a very common condition. However, various researchers have arrived at different figures and some have found that up to 20 per cent of children have the condition whereas others have suggested that 3 per cent of the childhood population has ADD.

These variations reflect the different criteria used by these workers in defining ADD. The true figure is somewhere between these two extremes and it certainly affects at least 5% of the childhood population

Children from all cultures and countries can be affected by the condition. ADD is seen more commonly in children with learning disabilities, conduct disorder, antisocial personality and Tourette Syndrome than other children.

Chapter 3 : About Attention Deficit Disorder

ADD is diagnosed about 3 to 10 times more often in boys than in girls. This is partly explained by the fact that ADD is easier to identify in boys because they tend to be more aggressive and are less able to control their impulses and activity levels than girls. It is much easier to spot significant behaviour problems, usually found in boys, than problems with attention in quiet children.

It is interesting that the same number of adult women and men have ADD. In other words, it is likely that the boys with ADD(+H) often 'outgrow' their more hyperactive, aggressive and impulsive traits in their teens but continue to experience various difficulties as a result of their ADD, particularly problems in paying attention.

Is Attention Deficit Disorder A New Condition ?

Although children with ADD have been on the scene for centuries, the condition is often not recognised for what it really is. Some medical, psychology and teaching professionals may not be aware that ADD exists. Others may deny that it exists, or they may brush the matter aside by making comments such as 'it's the flavour of the month' or 'ADD is a just passing fad'.

The classic and typical symptoms of ADD are sometimes passed off by some professionals as behavioural problems, learning disabilities or 'a phase he is going through, and which he'll grow out of'. Some people may even blame the parents for their 'poor parenting'. As a result, the diagnosis of ADD is sometimes missed.

Furthermore, ADD has been called many different names by many different people over the years. These different terms have created confusion among people even though they are talking about the same child.

Labels used by different workers have included: hyperactivity; dyslexia; hyperkinetic impulse disorder; minimal cerebral dysfunction; minimal brain damage; the hyperactive child syndrome; hyperkinetic reaction of childhood; behaviour disinhibition disorder; minimal cerebral palsy; attention deficit disorder; and attention deficit hyperactivity disorder.

Chapter 3 : About Attention Deficit Disorder

Because ADD is often poorly understood, ineffective and unsuitable treatments may be offered to families. Some of these methods may have been carried out over several months, or even years, at considerable financial hardship and emotional cost to the family.

Perhaps even more destructive is the attitude of non-believers. These may be friends, professionals or family members who deny that ADD exists. There are others who blame the child with ADD or his family for those problems that are really outside their control. Some people have a bias against various types of treatment, particularly the use of medications, as a result of their poor understanding of ADD and its management.

CHAPTER 4

THE TEMPERAMENT OF CHILDREN WITH ATTENTION DEFICIT DISORDER

> **Summary**
>
> Children with ADD(+H) are inclined to be demanding, impatient, immature, domineering, and easily frustrated.
>
> Those with ADD(-H) tend to be shy, sensitive and passive.
>
> All children with ADD share some common temperamental styles. They tend to be disorganised and unmotivated. They often put off making decisions and suffer from poor self-esteem.

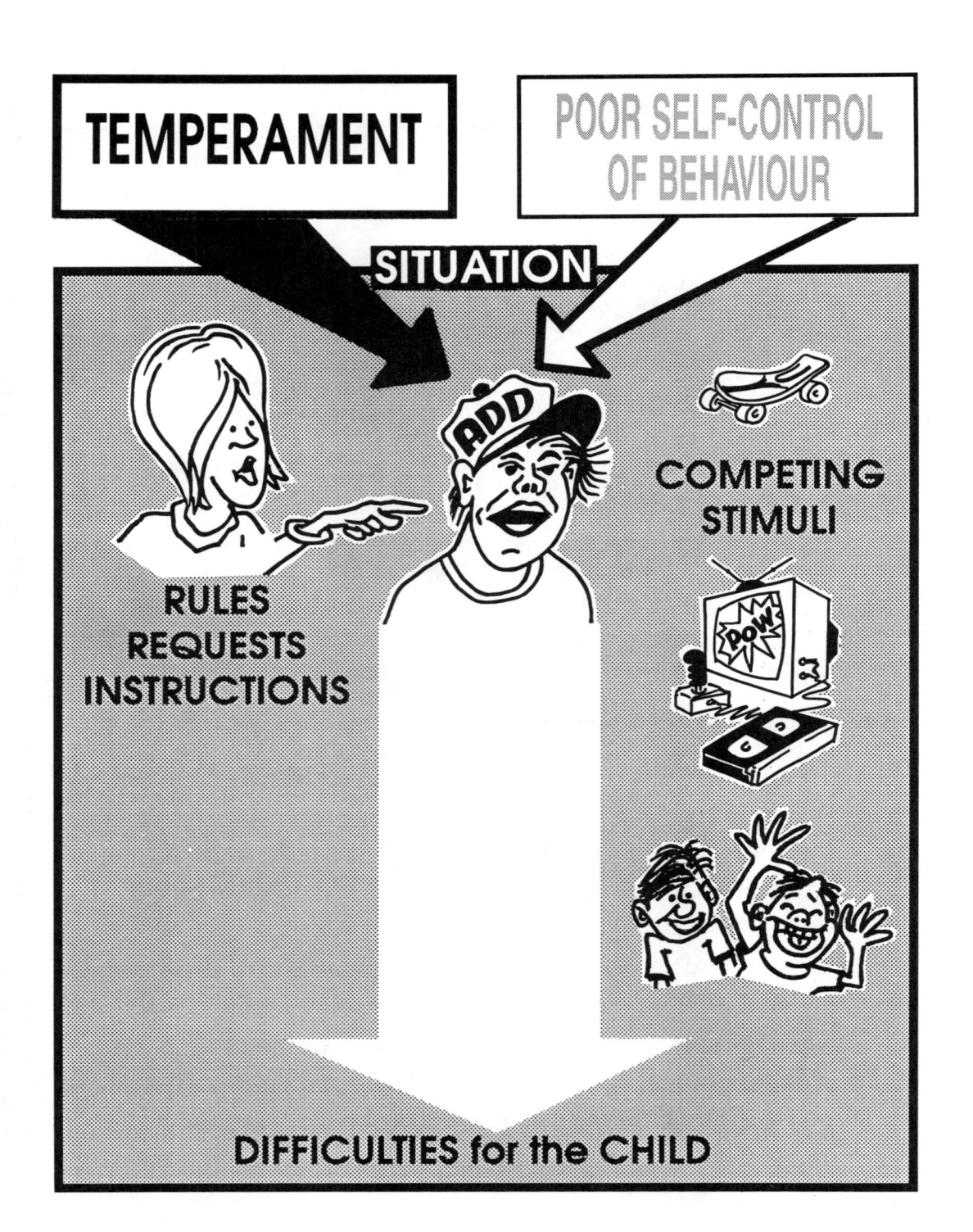

Chapter 4 : The Temperament Of Children With Attention Deficit Disorder

TEMPERAMENT

POOR SELF-CONTROL OF BEHAVIOUR

SITUATION

**RULES
REQUESTS
INSTRUCTIONS**

COMPETING STIMULI

DIFFICULTIES for the CHILD

Chapter 4 : The Temperament Of Children With Attention Deficit Disorder

About Temperament

Our temperament is a very important part of our identity. It is our individual make-up, personality or general style of operating and coping emotionally with different people and different situations. Many children with ADD have a make-up which makes it more difficult for them to control their behaviour and handle different situations. It also affects the way other people interact with them.

Children with ADD(+H) usually have a temperament which is very different from those with ADD(-H) and those who do not suffer from ADD. It is the interaction between the specific temperament style and difficulties in regulating behaviour which results in the typical characteristics of children with each type of ADD.

Temperament Of Children With ADD(+H) When They Were Young

Many, but not all, children who are later diagnosed as suffering from ADD(+H) are often described by their parents as being 'difficult' when they were very young.

His mother may have noticed that he was very active in the womb during the pregnancy. He was likely to have been a very active baby and toddler, and this included restlessness even when he was asleep. He did not need much sleep, woke in the early hours of the morning and he may have been a fussy feeder.

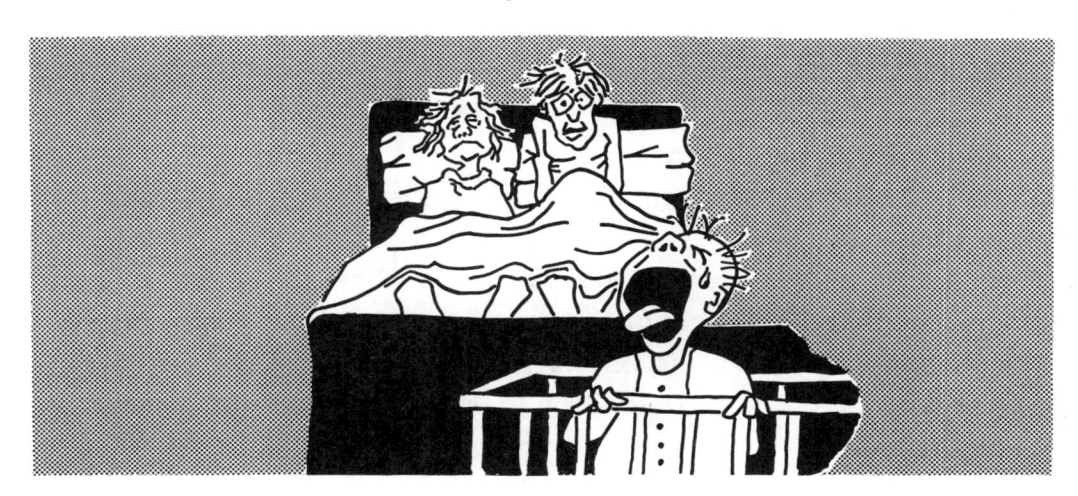

Chapter 4 : The Temperament Of Children With Attention Deficit Disorder

He was likely to have been irritable, colicky and difficult to cuddle. He had a tendency to cry a great deal and was very demanding and difficult to settle.

Such ongoing daily problems may have created great stress for the parents who questioned their parenting skills and lost their confidence and self-esteem. They may have consulted with various doctors and other specialists because they knew that something was 'wrong', but they were reassured that there was nothing to worry about. Although the parents may have tried various methods to calm him, nothing was really useful in helping them cope with their very stressful and frustrating situation. They may have been told that 'he will grow out of it' or perhaps they were labelled as being 'neurotic parents'.

Temperament Of Children With ADD(+H)

As he grows, the child with ADD(+H) often shows a particular style of conducting himself. He tends to be impatient and is unable to wait his turn in games and other activities. He finds it difficult to pursue and persist with long-term goals and activities requiring effort. He has problems in delaying gratification, lives in the here and now and is greatly influenced by what is happening around him.

He demands constant attention and approval. He also needs to be rewarded immediately and repeatedly because of his insatiability or difficulty in being kept satisfied. He is less likely to be aware of social rules and manners than other children. He is prone to overreact to criticism or correction and responds in an exaggerated and emotional way to comments made by other people. He may not respect the rights of others and is inclined to interfere in their activities.

He is inclined to be self-centred. He is preoccupied with himself and his own desires. He puts his own needs and wishes first, often involving himself in self-satisfaction and self-indulgence. These traits prompt people to label him as being selfish. His tendency to be inflexible and stubborn can lead to a variety of problems in relating to other people who may find it difficult to cope with his insistence that things have to be done his way. He carries out activities in his own particular manner and is unwilling to listen to or try alternatives suggested by other people.

Chapter 4 : The Temperament Of Children With Attention Deficit Disorder

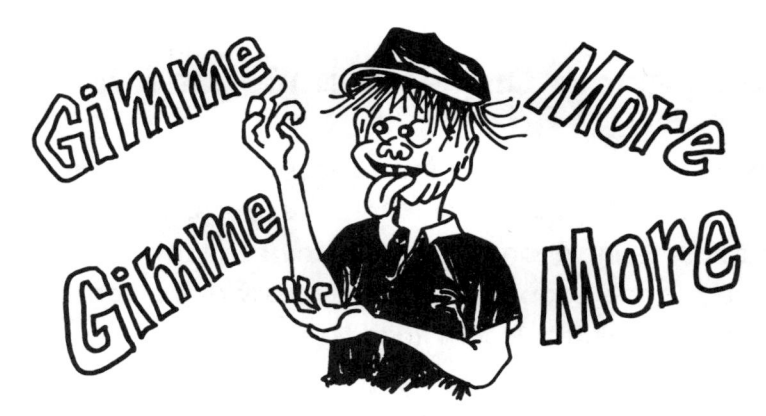

Because of his immature and naive nature, he is apt to be easily led and influenced by others. Alternatively he may attempt to dominate other children or even his parents. He is inclined to complain or blame other people for his own unacceptable behaviour, and he may deny that he actually carried out the behaviour in question. His frustration tolerance is rather low and he often reacts in an aggressive or negative way when things don't work out his way.

His parents may complain about difficulties he experiences in some of his daily habits. They may be concerned about his restlessness at night and poor sleep patterns including: talking in his sleep; night terrors; difficulty in falling asleep; frequent waking at night; or waking early in the morning. His appetite may also be affected and he may either be a fussy eater or have an increased appetite.

He is reluctant to accept change and because of this he manages far better with a regular routine. He is likely to have difficulties in coping with changes to his routine and when there are transitions in his activities.

Difficulties in the ability to organise himself can create a range of problems for him at home and at school. His tendency to procrastinate makes it difficult for him to make necessary choices and decisions and he often leaves things to the last minute.

He often lacks motivation to do things that need to be done. Because he is not a self-starter, he has to be constantly encouraged or even pushed by others, particularly his parents and teachers, to carry out various tasks.

Poor self esteem is a very common problem for the child with ADD(+H).

Chapter 4 : The Temperament Of Children With Attention Deficit Disorder

Consequences Of These Temperamental Traits

These temperamental traits may result in various unfortunate consequences for the child with ADD(+H). For instance his parents, brothers, sisters and teachers are likely to become increasingly frustrated by his incessant demands. As a result, he is likely to feel scapegoated, particularly as he cannot understand that he is the main contributor to their frustrations.

His feelings are often easily hurt and he may feel rejected by other people. This makes him more prone to blame them for causing his social isolation and for not caring about him. He may be labelled by others as being 'irresponsible', 'childish', 'rude', 'selfish', 'stubborn', 'disruptive' or 'inconsiderate'.

His 'difficult' temperament may greatly contribute to the stress experienced by his parents and teachers. These adults may view him as a 'problem' and after months of trying the usual types of discipline methods, they often respond by using more demanding and aggressive tactics in an attempt to change his 'attitude'. This may make the situation worse and a negative downward spiral may result, as the relationship between the child and the parents deteriorates.

Temperament Of Children With ADD(-H)

The child with ADD(-H) was likely to have been placid and relatively easy to get on with as a baby and toddler.

As a child he tends to be timid, withdrawn and shy and tends to keep to himself. His sensitivity and preoccupation with himself makes him reluctant to become involved in group activities, and he may seem to be detached and isolated from others. He tends to be passive, cooperative and compliant.

Although these characteristics are very different from ADD(+H), he shares some important traits with the child with ADD(+H). The child with ADD(-H) is also likely to procrastinate and may have difficulties with motivation. He is inclined to be very disorganised and experience poor self-esteem and a lack of confidence.

Chapter 4 : The Temperament Of Children With Attention Deficit Disorder

The diagnosis of ADD(-H) may be missed because he does not exhibit the more obvious hyperactive, 'difficult', intrusive and disruptive behaviour of the child with ADD(+H). However, some people may find his presence to be rather awkward and frustrating because he may be seen by them as being far too quiet, and because he does not become involved in their various activities. If this pattern persists, some people may stop trying to bring him out of his shell, and his poor self-esteem may deteriorate even further.

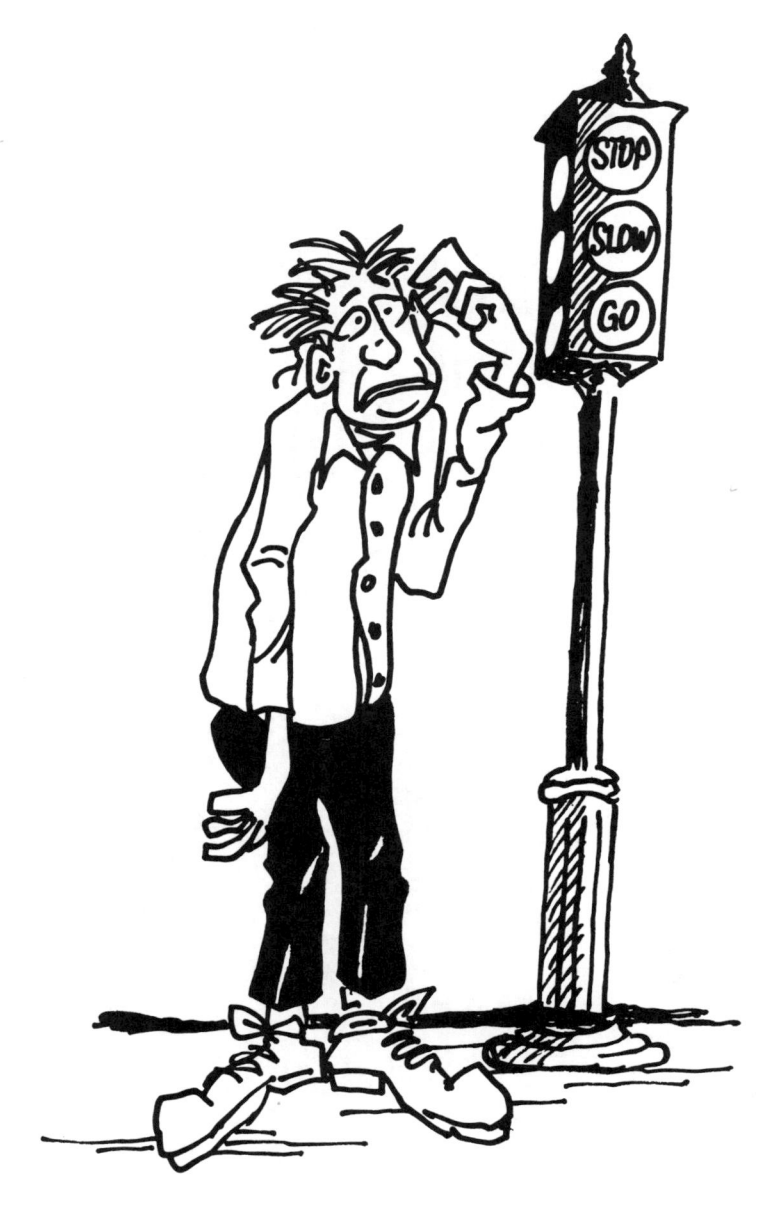

CHAPTER 5

THE BEHAVIOURS OF CHILDREN WITH ATTENTION DEFICIT DISORDER

Summary

His poor self-control of behaviour affects his ability to carry out various tasks.

He has difficulties in responding to rules and requests, especially in the presence of competing stimuli which are more powerful than the given instruction.

His behaviour varies a great deal and it is often unpredictable. It is influenced by other stimuli in his immediate environment.

His poor motivation can be a problem in some areas. He is less responsive to the usual incentives and rewards that are likely to motivate other children.

His performance and effort on various tasks are often inconsistent and erratic.

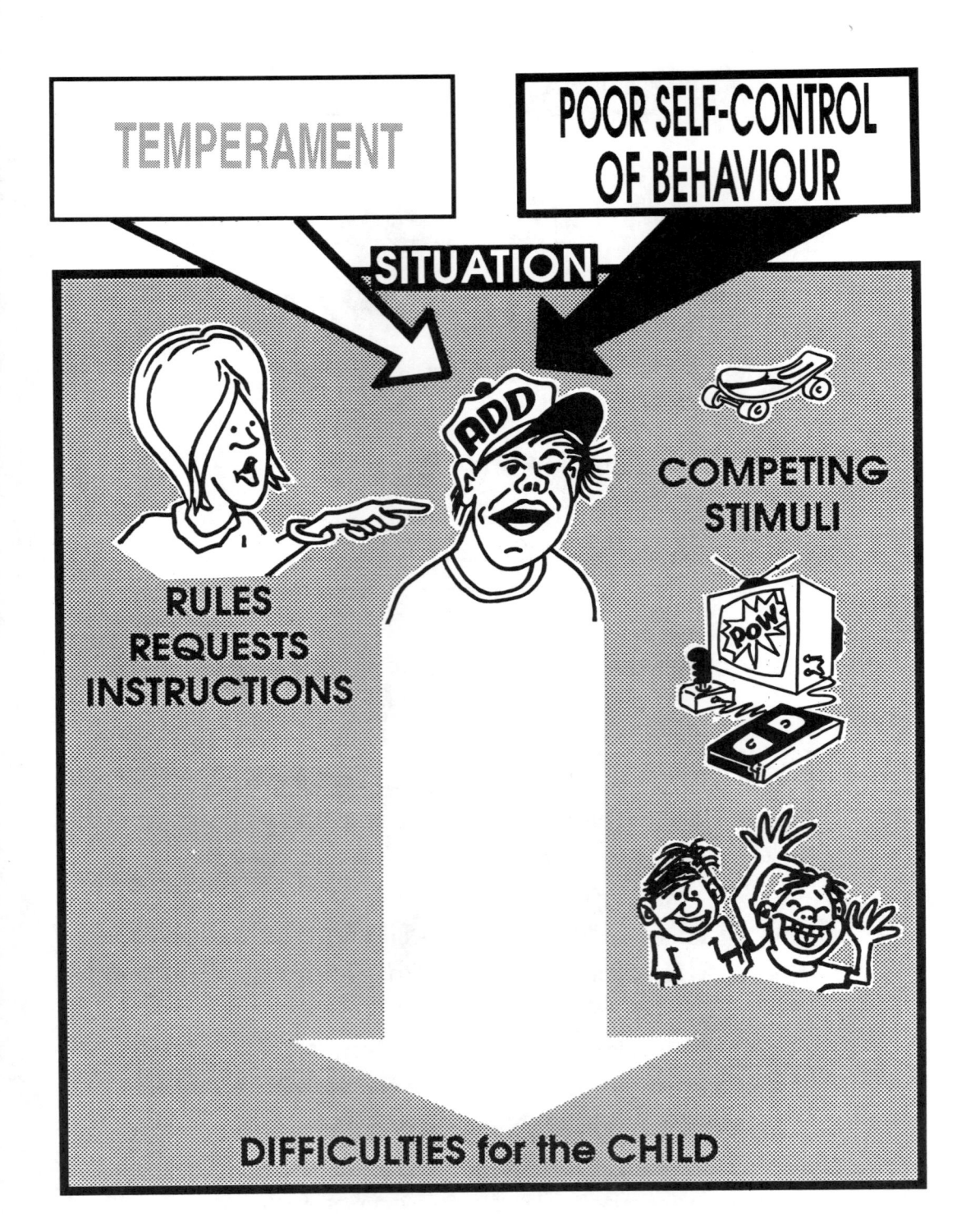

Chapter 5 : The Behaviours Of Children With Attention Deficit Disorder

TEMPERAMENT

POOR SELF-CONTROL OF BEHAVIOUR

SITUATION

RULES
REQUESTS
INSTRUCTIONS

COMPETING STIMULI

DIFFICULTIES for the CHILD

Chapter 5 : The Behaviours Of Children With Attention Deficit Disorder

Elements Of Behaviour In Children With ADD

Because the area of the brain which regulates self-control of behaviour does not operate in an efficient way, the child with ADD is likely to experience a wide variety of problems. These include:

- **Poor selective attention** or difficulty in focusing attention on the most relevant matter

- **Poor sustained attention** or trouble in continuing this focus over time

- **Difficulty in rejecting or blocking out distractions** and unnecessary stimuli

- **Poor interpretation of information** or problems in understanding the meaning of information and what is being said. This is the result of the difficulties he experiences in paying attention

- **Difficulty in setting goals**

- **Poor planning and a poor ability to organise himself**. This results in difficulties for him when it comes to working out the steps and materials needed to achieve certain goals

- **Difficulty in starting or initiating** necessary and important tasks or activities

- **Poor regulation of behaviour** and a reduced ability to check and modify what needs to be done

- **Lack of persistence** or difficulty in sustaining effort and in sticking at tasks

- **Difficulties in completing tasks, projects or activities**

These elements of behaviour are described in greater detail in Appendix 1: 'Specific Behavioural Aspects Of ADD'.

Daily Behaviours And Tasks

These obstacles in controlling behaviour may result in several problems. They influence the way in which he carries out various tasks and activities, and also in the way he feels and relates to people.

Chapter 5 : The Behaviours Of Children With Attention Deficit Disorder

He may have difficulties in carrying out routine tasks such as getting up in the morning; getting dressed; going to school; performing schoolwork, homework, projects or assignments; eating meals and carrying out house chores. He may not be 'with it' first thing in the morning. Because of his problems in planning and organisation, he may spend too much time in the shower or else find it difficult to locate the clothes and equipment needed for school. He often leaves things to the last minute and he is repeatedly running late for school.

Because of the problems with focusing and sustaining attention, he is likely to experience difficulties in learning, and so miss out on the important information and items required for homework. His difficulty in blocking out unimportant and distracting stimuli is often interpreted as 'being distracted'.

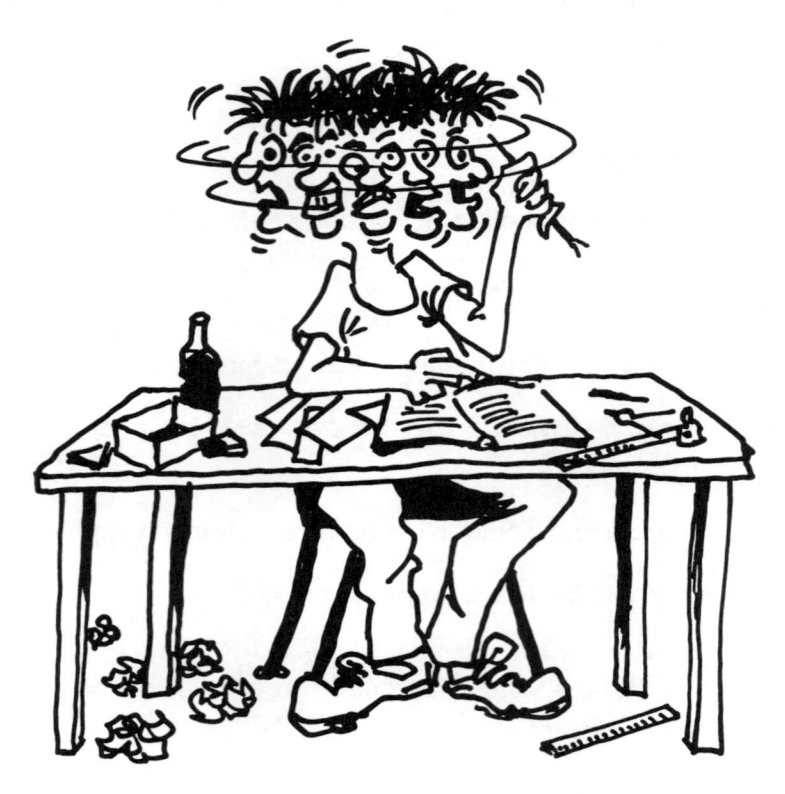

It may take him a long time to get started on important tasks. In any case, he may not fully understand what needs to be done because he has missed out on instructions given by his parents or teachers. His difficulty with persistence of effort, particularly on tasks requiring sustained attention, often results in 'mental burnout' and giving up. As a result, he often starts many activities but he has difficulty in completing them.

Chapter 5 : The Behaviours Of Children With Attention Deficit Disorder

He may also have difficulties in mastering special skills involved in recreational activities, hobbies, sport, study, solving problems and making plans. Each of these skills requires self-motivation, selective and sustained attention, practice, patience, repetition and persistence of effort. Problems in any of these areas may result in poor acquisition of skills, even though he may have the potential to do well. His difficulties with basic behavioural control may repeatedly let him down, in spite of his good intentions.

Because of poor control of muscle activity he may be very active and fidgety, and his writing and drawing may be untidy or even illegible at times. People may think that he is clumsy or accident prone. Although this may be partly the result of poor muscle control, it may be also explained by his poor selective attention on the important task at hand. His lapses in focus may result in 'silly' errors, untidy writing or in walking into a wall or tree because something else attracted his attention. Yet, at other times his coordination is excellent and he may sit almost perfectly still when he is focused on an interesting activity such as a television program, a computer game or his favourite hobby or pastime.

As a result of the problems in controlling his feelings and emotions, his moods may fluctuate and change quickly and noticeably. For instance, he may be happy for a while and when things are going right; then, with little provocation, he may become quite withdrawn and unhappy; next, he could become frustrated with a minor incident and launch immediately into a burst of anger or a rage attack; and this may be followed by remorse and guilt for having had a temper tantrum and upsetting others. He often cannot understand why he has such mood swings.

Chapter 5 : The Behaviours Of Children With Attention Deficit Disorder

His interactions with other people and other aspects of social behaviour may also create problems. He is less likely to pay attention to social cues and subtle messages from others, including family members, school mates and teachers. His mood swings, immaturity and demanding nature make it difficult for others to understand why he behaves poorly in social situations. He is often at a loss to understand how his own behaviour affects others.

Features Of General Behaviour In Children With ADD

The behaviour of the child with ADD(+H) can alter a great deal. This fact is very important and explains why it is so common to hear differing opinions about his behaviour from different people. In some situations he behaves in ways that are indistinguishable from other children. However, at different times and in different settings his behaviour may be very different, to the point of being deviant in the truest sense of the word.

His behaviour can be greatly influenced by the situation in which he finds himself and the task at hand. People may have great difficulty believing that he is almost angelic with his grandparents who, by the way, are likely to give him one-to-one attention and place very few demands on him. Yet he may be very aggressive and oppositional with his mother, the person who regularly gives him various instructions, thereby placing pressures and demands on him. These tax his ability in controlling his behaviour.

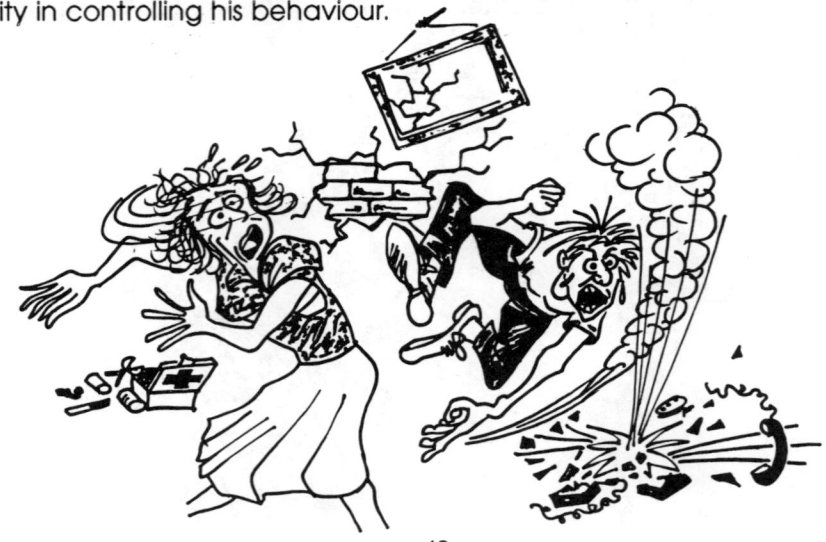

Chapter 5 : The Behaviours Of Children With Attention Deficit Disorder

There is frequently an uncertainty about his behaviour and other people often find it difficult to predict what he is going to do next. His behaviour can fluctuate greatly from moment to moment and, as a result, he may be described as being irresponsible, immature or dangerous. This finding applies particularly to the child with ADD(+H).

His efforts, performance and achievement in carrying out tasks are often erratic and inconsistent. He is capable of performing a particular task very well on one occasion, but he may carry out the very same task poorly a short time later. This results in stress and frustration for his parents, teachers and also himself. He may be considered 'lazy' because other people know that he can perform well, and they may wrongly conclude that he is refusing to repeat his good performance. Unfortunately, they are likely to be unaware of his difficulty with self-motivation. This erratic performance is common to children with ADD(+H) and ADD(-H).

Poor self-motivation is often a major problem for the child with ADD. He often needs to be motivated by other people in order to get him started on tasks and to persist with them. He needs to be encouraged frequently and also requires powerful incentives to spur him on. Difficulties with motivation apply to children with both types of ADD.

Variable Behaviour

His variable behaviour and performance can be a great source of frustration and concern for himself and his parents, teachers and other children. Because his concentration, behaviour and performance can vary greatly, teachers need to determine those situations and incentives which enable him to perform to the best of his ability.

It also means that the results of intelligence and achievement tests need to be interpreted with great caution because he can perform well sometimes but do poorly on other occasions. This applies to special 'once off' situations such as psychological testing and other assessment procedures in which he may do very well because of the novel situation and in which he receives individual attention. However, he may perform similar tasks badly in the classroom.

Chapter 5 : The Behaviours Of Children With Attention Deficit Disorder

In some situations his poor selective and sustained attention let him down and his recollection about specific matters can be very spotty and confused. He may be able to carry out the early steps of a task very well, but he may then make errors in later steps of the same task. He is often thought to be careless, but his errors are really the result of his problems in focusing and sustaining his attention on those tasks which require effort.

He is liable to give incorrect answers when required to carry out tasks involving memory. He can be at a considerable disadvantage in certain tasks such as tests and examinations and he is likely to make careless errors in spelling and arithmetic calculations.

The outcomes of his variable behaviour can be very significant. He may often make sincere and repeated promises to perform better but his good intentions often fail. These problems in poor self-control of behaviour may result in various different emotional reactions. For example, if he is repeatedly criticised or scolded for his various transgressions and mistakes, he may feel humiliated and inferior to others. He experiences embarrassment and probably resents his parents and teachers when they make an issue of his difficulties in controlling his behaviour or his poor academic progress. He is very likely to feel helpless and powerless. His vulnerable self-esteem will almost certainly deteriorate with the passage of time. This aggravates his existing difficulties.

Motivation And Incentives

He is less responsive than other children to requests, instructions or rules. Also, the usual rewards that work as incentives for other children are less likely to be powerful enough for him. This is more of a problem if an instruction is given in the presence of activities which are more interesting and stimulating than the given instruction itself. For example he is less likely to comply with a request to tidy his room if he is watching his favourite television program.

Because he is not a self-starter, he needs to be constantly motivated by other people. The challenge for his parents and teachers is to find better and more stimulating ways to encourage him to cooperate and carry out given tasks.

Chapter 5 : The Behaviours Of Children With Attention Deficit Disorder

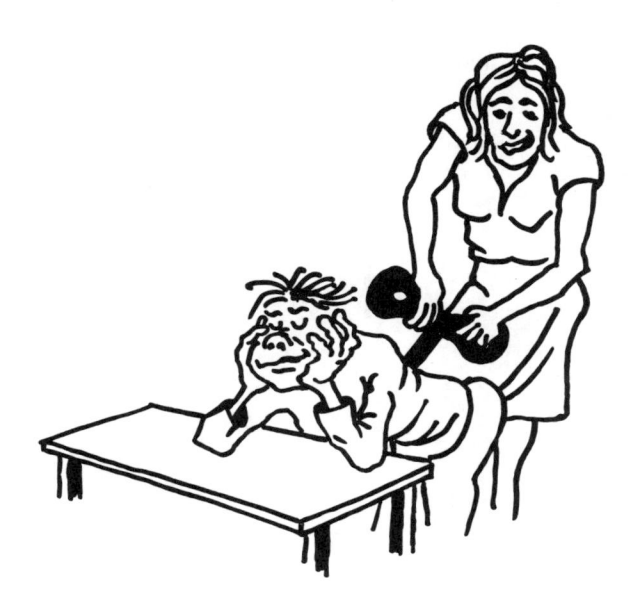

He often needs to be closely supervised in order to keep him on task and so that he carries through and completes the assigned activity. In other words, he has difficulties in following rules because his behaviour is greatly influenced by other more stimulating things in the immediate environment, and the instruction may become immaterial and unimportant for him. This may be easily mistaken by his parents and teachers as disobedience, and they are likely to become frustrated because of his lack of cooperation and compliance.

He is, however, more likely to carry out a request if the consequence matters to him. As a result of this, incentives and consequences need to be interesting, relevant and important to him. His efforts need to be rewarded immediately after the task has been carried out because he is insatiable and lacks patience. He lives in the here and now. Any delay in giving consequences or rewards for his behaviour is likely to be of little value.

Since he is less sensitive to incentives than other children, he loses interest in rewards more quickly than other children. He becomes quickly habituated to them and boredom sets in rapidly with the use of the same reward if it is offered repeatedly. Incentives therefore need to be changed or rotated frequently in order to help motivate him.

Chapter 6: Different Situations - Different Behaviours

CHAPTER 6

DIFFERENT SITUATIONS - DIFFERENT BEHAVIOURS

Summary

Although ADD has a physiologic basis, his behaviour and attention are greatly influenced by factors in his immediate environment.

There are some situations which enable him to enhance his self-control, and enable him to improve his performance and behaviour.

Other situations may tax his self-control and these may create difficulties for him in controlling his behaviour and attention.

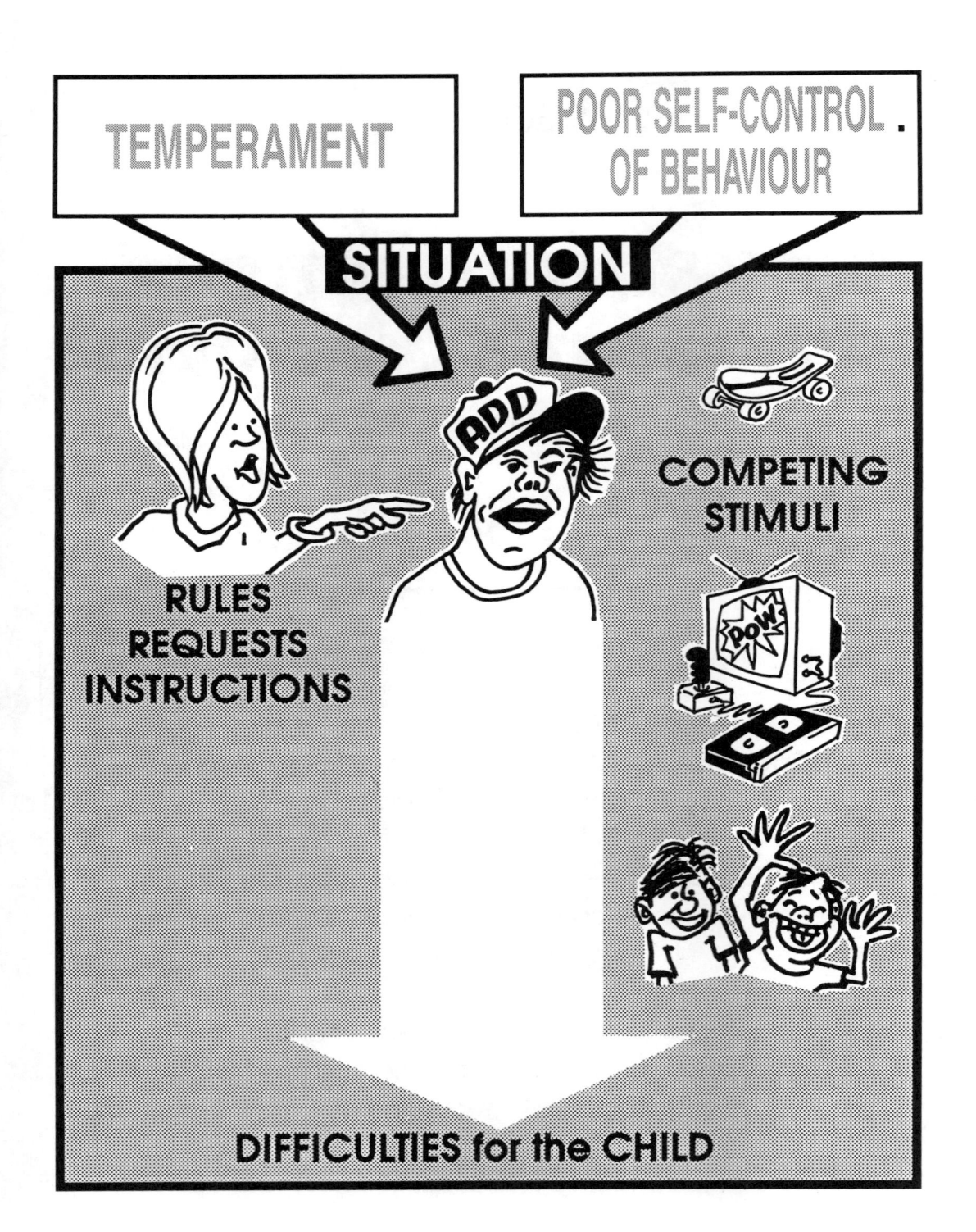

Chapter 6: Different Situations - Different Behaviours

TEMPERAMENT

POOR SELF-CONTROL OF BEHAVIOUR

SITUATION

RULES
REQUESTS
INSTRUCTIONS

COMPETING STIMULI

DIFFICULTIES for the CHILD

Chapter 6: Different Situations - Different Behaviours

Some General Comments

The effect of different situations on the child with ADD can be better understood if we take into account some important factors. He often suffers from mental fatigue and has greater difficulties with his poor self-control in the late afternoon and evenings. This 'mental burnout' can result in various problems in controlling behaviour, careless errors and poor quality of work.

His mother is likely to experience more difficulties with his behaviour than his father because she usually has more contact with him and is therefore more likely to impose more demands, requests and instructions. It is often difficult to keep him satisfied and he tends to become easily bored. He finds it difficult to block out irrelevant and unimportant stimuli which compete with tasks that need to be carried out.

Creating structure in his environment improves his self-control and enables him to cope better. When the amount of stimulation is too great, however, he is more prone to experience difficulties in controlling his behaviour and attention. He often finds it difficult to cope with changes in his routine and during transitions from one activity to another.

He constantly seeks one-to-one attention and when this is not forthcoming his control is likely to deteriorate. Alternatively, he may seek such attention, often using demanding tactics to get it. This is why he often finds it difficult to manage his behaviour in a group situation.

He needs to be given frequent and powerful incentives and rewards in order to keep him motivated. If these are not forthcoming, he may become bored, his attention wanders and his behaviour is likely to deteriorate.

He frequently searches for something more stimulating than the task at hand, particularly if the task lacks sufficient interest or is too difficult for him. Television and computer games are stimulating and enjoyable and they often hold his attention extremely well. In a similar way, favourite hobbies and pastimes often take precedence over house chores or homework.

Chapter 6: Different Situations - Different Behaviours

Situational Variables

The symptoms of ADD often vary a great deal from time to time and from place to place. The important temperamental and behavioural variables of children with ADD have already been discussed.

Some situations and settings can accommodate his difficulties with self-control whereas others place greater demands on his temperamental style as well as his behavioural and motivational problems. It is important to realise this so that appropriate modifications may be made to his different environments and so provide him with a better opportunity to function more effectively.

All situations have a variety of competing stimuli such as people, activities, furniture, materials and objects of different colours and textures, sounds and visual stimuli, activities and a range of other potential distractions. Any of these may be interpreted by the child with ADD as being either stimulating or boring.

Situations Which Are Less Troublesome For Children With ADD

His behaviour and attention are more likely to be within his control when there are few demands placed on him. He is very likely to cope better when he plays on his own, when allowed to do his 'own thing' and when washing or bathing.

He is often better behaved in the presence of his father who usually spends less time with him and gives fewer requests and instructions. His father is likely to be firmer and more assertive with him than his mother and this tends to improve his ability to cooperate and comply with instructions.

He usually experiences fewer problems when he receives immediate rewards and feedback for cooperating and complying with requests. In a very similar way, immediate consequences need to be given for any lack of cooperation so that he can keep on track and on task and so improve his ability to cope.

Chapter 6: Different Situations - Different Behaviours

His self-control improves when he is able to focus his attention on stimulating activities. This is why he is likely to enjoy watching television and perform well when using computers and playing with electronic games and with his favourite hobbies. His attention and behaviour are better when instructions are repeated and when he receives one-to-one attention. Structured situations tend to keep him more focused, but these also need to be stimulating and colourful.

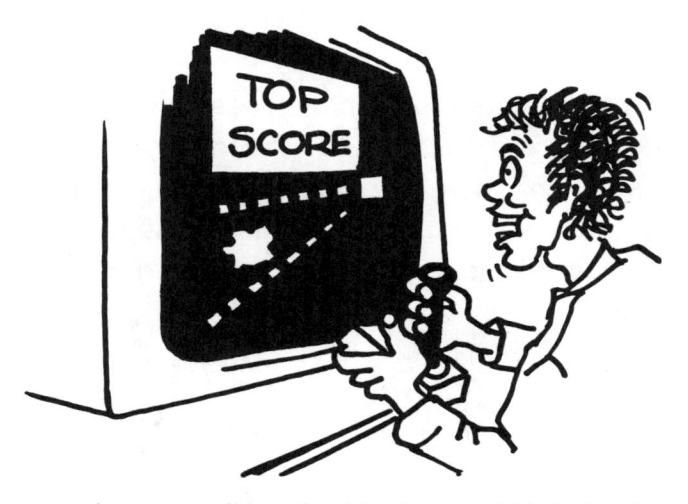

The time of day can be a very important factor, and his behaviour and attention is often much better from mid-morning through to mid-afternoon, and before mental burnout occurs.

He is likely to cope better in new or unfamiliar situations because his insatiability is less of a problem in such settings. This explains why infrequent visits to his grandparents or starting at a new school are less likely to create difficulties for him initially. However, after repeated exposures, the novelty wears off and he is likely to become habituated to these situations and difficulties are more likely to be experienced.

Situations Which Are More Troublesome For Children With ADD

There are some situations which are likely to create obstacles for him since they are likely to tax his difficulties with motivation, behaviour control and in paying attention.

Chapter 6: Different Situations - Different Behaviours

He is quite likely to experience difficulties in the more familiar situations, most often home and school. These settings are often perceived as non stimulating or 'boring' places in which a variety of demands are imposed on him. It is usually his mother and teachers who repeatedly give instructions and request that he carries out various tasks. They are the people who attempt to gain his cooperation in carrying out schoolwork as well as chores and routines such as getting dressed, tidying his room and doing his homework.

Because of his insatiable nature and preference for one-to-one attention, he is more likely to experience difficulties with self-control of behaviour and attention in the following situations: when his parents are on the telephone; when visiting another person's home; when people visit his home; in public places such as supermarkets and restaurants; when playing with with a group of children; and in other group situations.

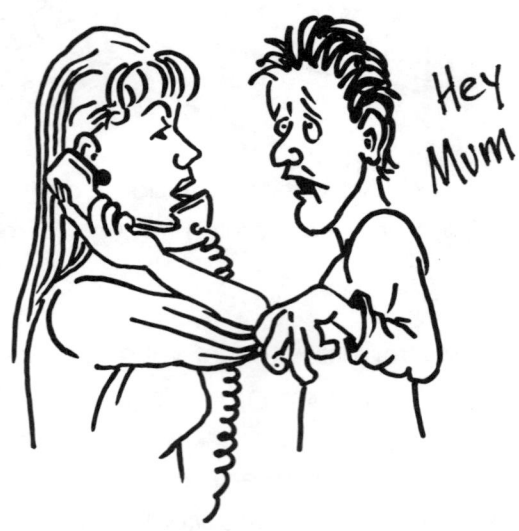

Situations which are boring or not stimulating often tax his difficulties in focusing and sustaining his attention and are likely to create problems for him. These include: situations in which he is not rewarded for the effort or performance he puts into tasks; performing tasks which require sustained attention at school, for example academic work; and those activities which demand a high level of planning and organising, for example homework and school projects. These tasks place additional demands on him because they require him to control his behaviour and activity level. His motivation and self-control are often problems for him first thing in the morning. His difficulties are often compounded in the late afternoon and evening hours when he is mentally or physically exhausted.

CHAPTER 7

CONDITIONS RELATED TO ATTENTION DEFICIT DISORDER

> **Summary**
>
> Other conditions can coexist with ADD.
>
> These include poor self-esteem,
> a range of developmental disabilities such as
> language, learning, muscle coordination disorders,
> and
> problems in controlling bladder and bowel function.
>
> ADD can masquerade as other conditions.

Chapter 7 : Conditions Related To Attention Deficit Disorder

Developmental Problems

When compared to the general population, children with ADD are at greater risk of suffering a range of other conditions which result from developmental immaturities. This is not really surprising because ADD is also a developmental problem. Any immaturity in one area of the brain is more likely to be associated with immaturities in other areas.

Some regions of the brain are involved in the understanding and processing of information and enable the child to learn important skills involving speech and language, various academic skills and coordinating muscle movement. Also, the brain regulates bladder and bowel control. If there are immaturities in the way these brain regions operate, it is quite likely that the child will experience difficulties in mastering these skills.

Although any of these developmental problems may occur independently, they are seen more commonly in children with ADD than in other children. It is important that the assessment of the child with ADD takes into account the possible coexistence of these conditions because they may require treatment in their own right. If only one condition is treated without considering the others, only a partial improvement of the overall situation will result.

General Comments About Developmental Problems

These developmental conditions tend to have an hereditary basis and it is not uncommon to find that a relative of the child has, or has had, similar problems. Some of these conditions may be identified in early life, particularly if they are severe. Some children may experience a mild disability only, whereas others may suffer from a moderate or severe problem.

All of these related problems may result in a range of emotional difficulties such as frustration, depression, avoidance of effort, underachievement and a sense of failure. His stress may show itself in a variety of behaviour problems such as defiant and aggressive behaviour, or as isolation and social withdrawal. Other people such as his parents and teachers may not understand the nature of his difficulties and they may label him as being lazy or poorly motivated.

Chapter 7 : Conditions Related To Attention Deficit Disorder

These conditions may occur in different combinations. For instance, one child may have mild ADD without any of the other possible associated conditions. Another child may suffer from moderate ADD together with a significant reading disorder. A third child may suffer from ADD and experience muscle coordination and language disorders and also poor self-esteem.

The outcomes of these disorders can vary, depending on the type of disorder, its severity and the age of the child at the time of diagnosis and when treatment was commenced. If the existence of any of these conditions is suspected, a proper assessment needs to be carried out before suitable treatment is begun. His coexisting ADD also needs to be treated appropriately in order to improve the overall outcome.

Poor Self-Esteem

It is thought that self-esteem is at least partly governed by the same area of the brain which is involved in regulating and controlling behaviour. Poor self-esteem often coexists with ADD. A child's poor self-esteem causes him to feel badly about himself and it may affect all facets of his life. It saps his confidence and is likely to result in negative emotions and attitudes about himself and a whole range of areas involving his life. It may also adversely affect the way he relates to various people in his life and how he carries out tasks and behaviours.

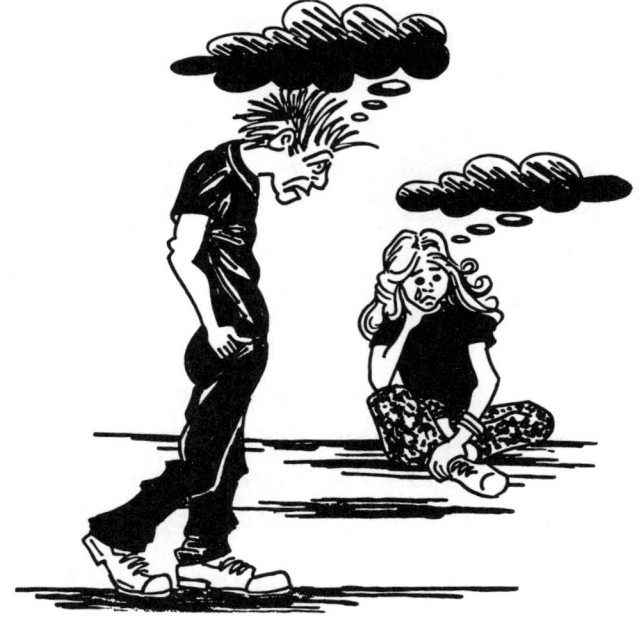

Chapter 7 : Conditions Related To Attention Deficit Disorder

Self-esteem can be also influenced by a range of psychological and social factors. The child with ADD often has a history of repeated poor performance and negative interactions with others over many years, and these are likely to aggravate his poor self-esteem.

Learning Disabilities

A variety of specific learning disabilities can occur together with ADD. These academic skills disorders include **reading disorder** which was once known as dyslexia, **writing disorder** and **arithmetic disorder.**

The crucial feature of **reading disorder** is his difficulty in understanding and interpreting written work. This results in underachievement in those areas which require the use of reading skills. His reading is likely to be slow and laboured and he often makes a variety of errors when attempting this skill.

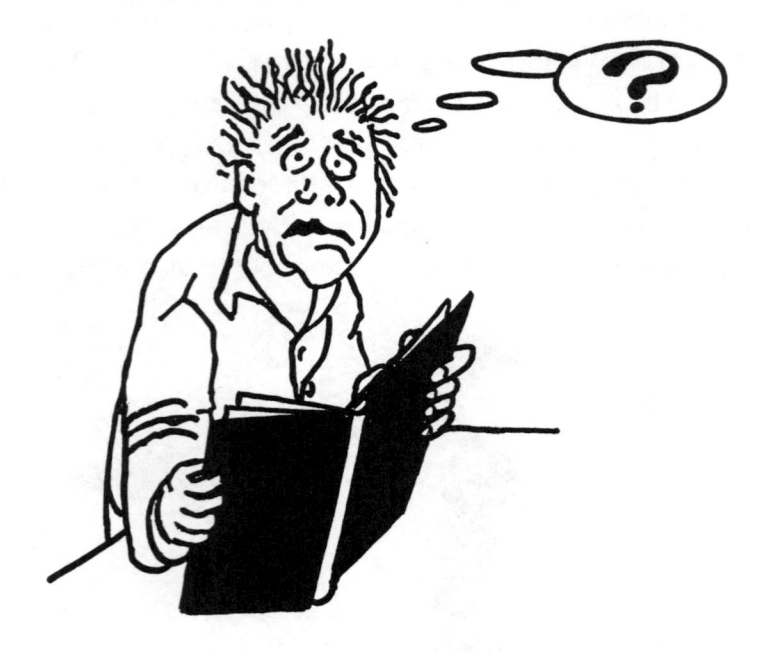

Writing disorder is recognised when he experiences significant difficulties in composing written work. It is frequently accompanied by errors in spelling, punctuation and grammar, and written work is often poorly organised. These problems result in underachievement in those subjects which depend on the correct use of written work.

Chapter 7 : Conditions Related To Attention Deficit Disorder

Arithmetic disorder is identified when he experiences substantial difficulties in carrying out a variety of arithmetic skills. There are a number of specific and related skills involved in mathematics including: understanding mathematical terms; understanding and processing mathematics symbols and operations such as addition, subtraction, division and multiplication; converting written words into mathematical symbols and signs; and grouping similar symbols into meaningful operations. Difficulties in using any of these skills are likely to result in great difficulties in managing daily activities which require the accurate use of these skills.

Language And Speech Disorders

There are a number of disorders which involve the development of language and speech. Some of the more common types will be briefly discussed. They may occur in various combinations.

Articulation disorder is suspected if he experiences repeated difficulties in using speech sounds in the correct way. For instance he may substitute one sound for another, leave out sounds from words or make the wrong sound. It may be a mild disability, in which case his speech may be totally intelligible; or else it can be severe to the point where it is very difficult for other people to understand what he is saying.

Expressive language disorder is the term applied to those children who experience a delay in the development of spoken language. It may result in: a limited range of vocabulary; poor acquisition of new vocabulary; errors in speech; poor grammar; and the omissions or disregard of important parts of speech.

Receptive language disorder refers to a significant delay in the development in the understanding of language spoken by other people. In some cases it only involves difficulties in understanding certain words or phrases. In more severe cases he may experience great difficulty in understanding simple sentences, in distinguishing the difference between sounds, in putting words into the correct sequence, and in the storage and recall of speech sounds.

Chapter 7 : Conditions Related To Attention Deficit Disorder

Coordination Disorder Or Motor Skills Disorder

Coordination disorder is suspected when he demonstrates a significant delay in the development of muscle skills. 'Clumsiness' is the term which is often used to describe this condition. There are three basic types of coordination difficulties and they may occur in various combinations.

Poor gross motor coordination refers to clumsiness involving the use of the large muscles and it is often seen as frequent tripping or difficulties in hopping and running.

Poor fine motor coordination is seen as clumsiness when the small muscles are used. It often results in difficulties in tying shoe laces or in buttoning.

Poor eye-hand and poor eye-foot coordination affects those activities that require the eyes and the hands or feet to work as a team. It is noticed as untidy handwriting and difficulties in catching or kicking a ball.

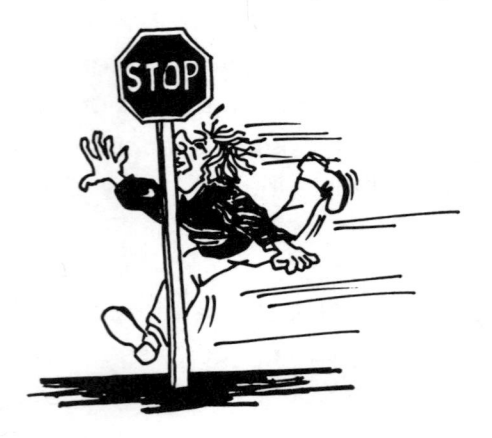

Bedwetting And Soiling

Enuresis is the term which refers to the repeated and unintentional passage of urine. The common type is bedwetting when urine is voided while he is asleep. Another type, diurnal enuresis, refers to the involuntary emptying of the bladder both during the day into his clothes and at night.

Encopresis refers to the involuntary passage of stools or faeces into his clothes.

Chapter 7 : Conditions Related To Attention Deficit Disorder

Tourette Syndrome

Tourette Syndrome is a neurological condition which usually presents itself as repeated, involuntary, sudden jerky or 'twitchy' movements, or tics, involving muscles of various parts of the body as well as the vocal organs which result in a variety of involuntary sounds and utterances. Many of the sufferers of Tourette Syndrome experience ADD as an associated feature.

Tourette Syndrome is also associated with a range of other conditions, some of which are shared with ADD. For example, people with Tourette Syndrome are at risk of also having obsessive compulsive disorder, mood disorders ('lows' or 'highs' or both), developmental disorders such as those mentioned above, panic attacks, a range of sleep disturbances, oppositional defiant disorder and conduct disorder.

A careful assessment of children with possible Tourette Syndrome is important because each of the various potential coexisting conditions may need to be treated in addition to the involuntary movements.

Oppositional And Aggressive Behaviours

The literature suggests that oppositional and aggressive behaviours are often associated with ADD, particularly in those children with ADD(+H). **Oppositional defiant disorder** and the more severe **conduct disorder** are more likely to be complications of ADD(+H) rather than conditions that are directly related to it.

Oppositional defiant disorder tends to show up in the older child or adolescent whose untreated ADD(+H) results in difficult and negative interactions between the child and other people over many years. These interactions often escalate and he reacts increasingly with defiant behaviour and verbal aggression.

Conduct disorder is a condition which is a more extreme form of aggression in which his antisocial behaviour infringes upon the rights of others.

These conditions will be discussed further in Chapter 15: 'The Future Of Children With Attention Deficit Disorder'.

Chapter 7 : Conditions Related To Attention Deficit Disorder

Attention Deficit Disorder - The Great Masquerader

ADD itself may mimic some of the disorders already described. Consider, for example, a child whose handwriting is untidy, particularly when he carries out this activity in a busy classroom. The impression to the casual observer may be that he has an eye-hand coordination problem. Yet, on closer observation it is noted that he can write quite neatly and accurately in a one-to-one situation when presented with an enjoyable topic. It is likely that his ADD masquerades as a muscle coordination problem, in that the untidy writing is really a reflection of problems in paying attention to the task and poor control of muscle activity in an environment which is distracting for him.

Once treatment of his ADD with medication is commenced, his handwriting may improve dramatically. This is the result of an improved ability to focus on tasks and persist in activities involving effort. These include handwriting. If he is not helped with such treatment, then there is a strong likelihood that a true fine motor coordination problem exists.

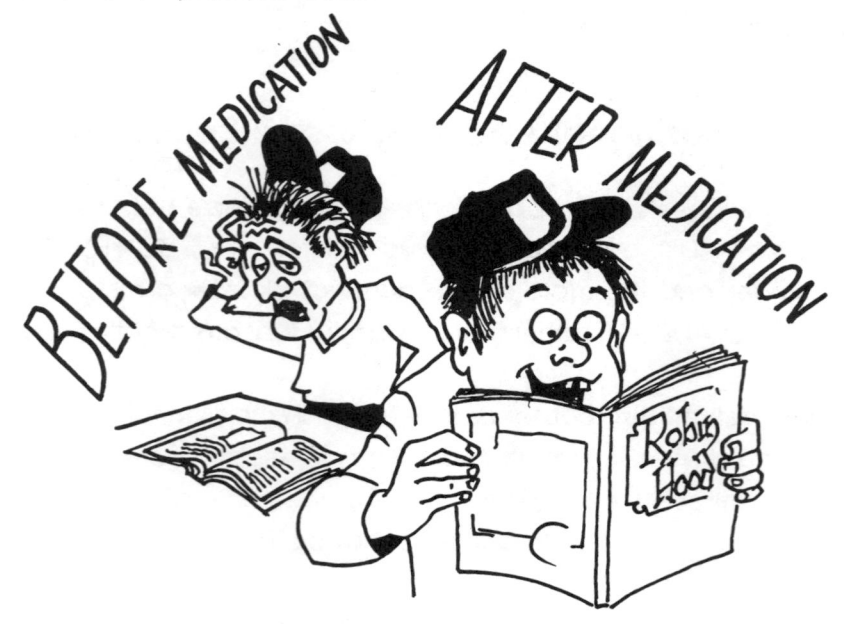

The same is true in the case of the child who is suspected of having a learning disability in, say, reading or spelling. He may be underachieving in these areas at school. However, his parents may notice that he is capable of performing very reasonable work in these areas, particularly in quiet one-to-one situations.

Chapter 7 : Conditions Related To Attention Deficit Disorder

Once the diagnosis of ADD is made and suitable treatment is instituted, he is often able to pay attention to tasks and persist with them. The rate of progress in his school work often improves dramatically. In other words, his problems with poor selective and sustained attention, resulting from his ADD, is the more likely reason for his underachievement. In other words, his ADD is masquerading as a specific learning disability.

It is important to consider the possibility of ADD in children who show evidence of any of the developmental problems mentioned above. ADD may be the major factor involved in the cause of a range of learning and related problems. Alternatively, ADD may be a contributory factor in the child's difficulties.

If the diagnosis of ADD is suspected, then it needs to be properly assessed and managed first - before the other diagnoses and conditions are considered. It is vital that the child's attention and behavioural difficulties are remedied before specific management for other conditions is introduced. If there is a possibility that any of the other conditions also exist, they need to be assessed on their own merits after treatment of the ADD has been started.

Chapter 8: Living With Attention Deficit Disorder

CHAPTER 8

LIVING WITH ATTENTION DEFICIT DISORDER

Summary

Children with ADD have a chronic disability and they often experience a range of difficulties in many areas of their lives.

They attempt to cope as best they can with their disability on a daily basis.

They also need to learn to cope with the negative reactions of other people who may not understand their disability.

They often exhibit many strengths which need to be encouraged.

Chapter 8 : Living With Attention Deficit Disorder

The Daily Plight Of Children With ADD

ADD can be a mild condition in many children whereas other children may be severely affected. A child with mild ADD often copes quite well and is able to carry out his daily activities without many difficulties. He may only need minimal treatment, perhaps medication, to help him focus and sustain his attention and control other minor difficulties.

The child with severe ADD may not be so fortunate. His condition may pose a number of major obstacles for him. For instance his problems in maintaining attention may result in significant learning problems and underachievement in various areas at school. His difficulties in controlling his behaviour are likely to create problems for him at home, at school and with his friends.

His situation may be even more complicated if any of the related conditions, for example poor self-esteem or a learning disability, are also present. He has to cope with many disadvantages and challenges which the condition imposes on him. His disability is with him day-in, day-out and there is no escape.

To make matters worse, the difficulties which he experiences are often poorly understood by his family, teachers and friends. He is forced to cope, in the best way he can, with their negative reactions. This is no mean feat for a child whose self-esteem may be already compromised and who is already experiencing great stress as a result of his disability. These are all very real concerns for him and they need to be considered when the assessment is carried out.

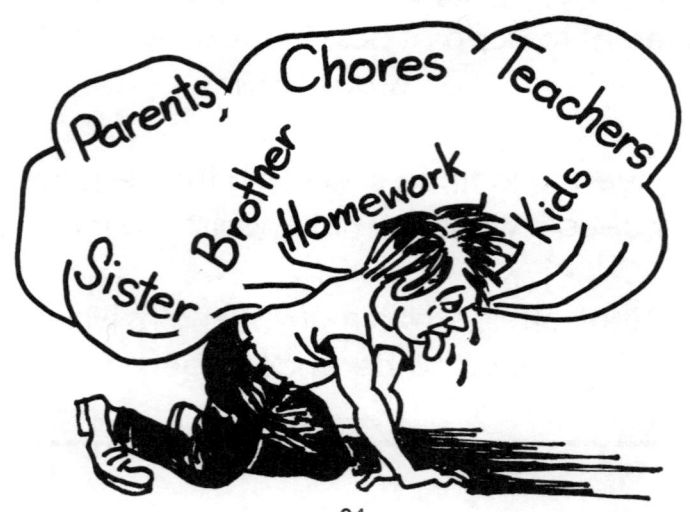

He may not understand why he behaves in the way he does and why other people treat him in negative ways. Although he may realise and feel that there is something amiss, he is usually at a loss to explain why. The people around him are often as baffled as he is.

The stress of living with ADD often results in a variety of emotional reactions. These include: anger, irritation and frustration; confusion, anxiety; disappointment; self-blame; feelings of persecution; and fears of certain situations. Stress may also result in headaches and many other psychosomatic symptoms.

The child who has ADD(+H), characterised by poor self-control of behaviour, may not understand why he is in constant trouble. Nor does he realise why he becomes very easily frustrated and frequently loses his temper at the slightest provocation.

Children with ADD are likely to experience some common reactions. These include: the frustration of being forgetful; feelings of uncertainty about both the immediate situation and about his future; knowing that he is 'different'; the fear that he is 'abnormal' or that there is something seriously wrong with him; the experience of stress and anxiety in a variety of different situations; the feelings of helplessness and inability to take control of his life; and difficulties in paying attention, being organised, and in starting and completing important tasks.

He is prone to suffer from poor self-esteem and often experiences a lack of confidence. Sometimes his parents wonder if he is depressed. He may suffer guilt and sometimes blames himself for creating problems for his family and other people in his life.

Labels

It is quite common that other people, out of sheer frustration, start using a variety of adverse and negative terms to describe him. These include: irresponsible; disruptive; stubborn; rude; immature; childish; selfish; careless; lazy; and stupid. The use of such labels is very unfortunate because they are likely to be quite demeaning and destructive. These people do not understand his difficulties.

These labels focus on his negative qualities and ignore his assets, abilities and potential. This 'blaming the victim' mentality is likely to hinder the introduction of suitable programs to help him overcome his difficulties. The practice of using labels can result in negative feelings which are likely to worsen his poor self-esteem and confidence. Once a label or 'bad reputation' has stuck, it is often very difficult to eradicate, even if there is significant progress in his behaviour.

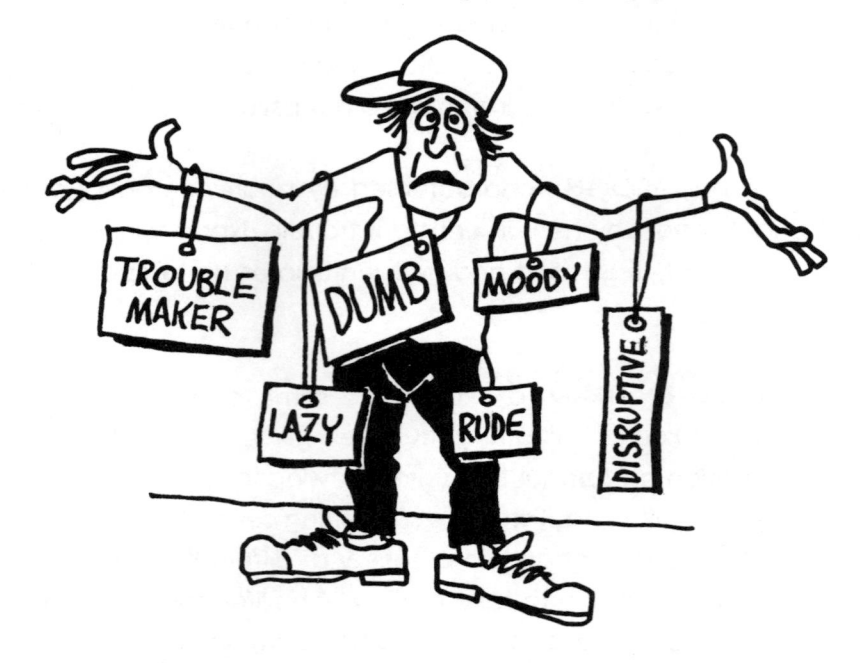

Labels tend to isolate him from others and they result in poor communication between other people and himself. Any label can produce and maintain a 'self-fulfilling prophecy', and if this occurs, he is likely to come to believe it and act accordingly. The use of negative terms reduces his capacity to change his behaviour in acceptable ways.

The Reactions Of Other People

His disability may provoke negative reactions from others including parents, brothers and sisters, other family members, teachers and other children. They are likely to be confused by his erratic behaviour, poor progress at school and the other difficulties he experiences. Many of their reactions are negative and could further damage his already fragile self-esteem.

Their reactions include overprotection and sympathy. He may be blamed and criticised for his behaviour and this could lead to disapproval, condemnation, constant reprimands and even rejection. Some people may humiliate him and others may retaliate in a physical manner. These reactions are often difficult to overcome. They can contribute to his social isolation and poor self-esteem. Not only is he at a constant disadvantage because of his ADD, but he also tries to cope and contend with the additional stress imposed by others.

Attention Deficit Disorder As A Strength

The child with ADD often possesses very positive and desirable qualities. These may be easily forgotten or overlooked because people, parents and teachers included, often focus on the negative features of his behaviour and personality.

He may be very talented and creative in fields such as computer work, writing and art. This is often accompanied by an active imagination and he is often very resourceful. He may be described as being loving and caring, particularly with younger children and animals. He can be a kind and generous friend.

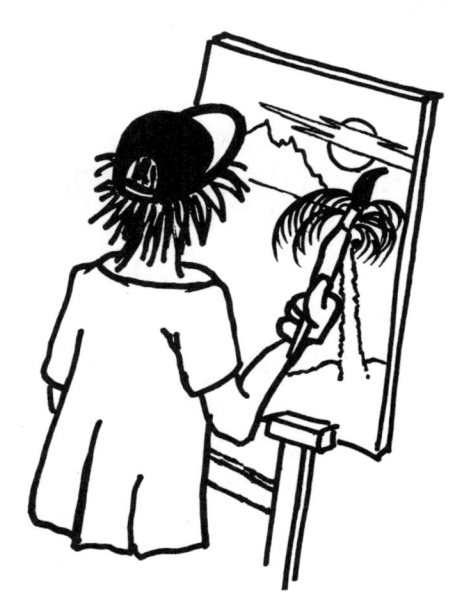

His energy, physical strength, athletic abilities, skills and playfulness enable him to become involved in many different pursuits which can result in excellent work in areas of interest such as hobbies and sport. His assertiveness and energetic style are great assets. He can be competitive, vigorous and ambitious, and his drive can be targeted to toward positive areas and pursuits. His intelligence provides him with the potential to perform well academically.

He may be a lateral thinker, sensitive and creative. These strengths may result in many great ideas as he uses his inquiring and inquisitive mind. He may be witty and humorous and his friendly and outgoing manner can be a great asset.

The child with ADD has great potential in many areas. The challenge for parents and teachers is to manage him in positive ways and encourage him to use his assets and strengths to advantage. In this way he can be guided in positive directions so that this potential is realised.

There are many successful people who suffered from ADD as children. They have excelled in many fields such as literature, medicine, acting, business, politics, sport, teaching, art, science and technology and many more. The list of famous people who performed well in spite of their disability includes: Albert Einstein; Winston Churchill; Ludwig van Beethoven; and Dustin Hoffman. The child with ADD can become successful in his selected fields of endeavour and his future is likely to be very positive if his condition is managed properly.

The Needs Of Children With ADD

He needs to understand all aspects of his condition and how it affects him. He must learn to accept that he has a disability. Such acceptance is a process which may take considerable time. The treating professional should explain these matters in an accurate, matter-of-fact and sensitive way and in language which he understands. The child should be encouraged to ask questions and clarify any matters which he does not understand.

The child with ADD needs to feel accepted by his family. His parents also need to be 'educated' about his ADD so they can understand the reasons for his difficulties with attention and behaviour control. They need to learn about the various forms of treatment available and the necessary special skills required to accommodate his disability.

CHAPTER 9

FAMILIES OF CHILDREN WITH ATTENTION DEFICIT DISORDER

> **Summary**
>
> Stress is common in the families of the child who has ADD.
>
> His ADD may contribute to difficulties in relationships between various members of the family.
>
> Other members of the family may suffer from a variety of psychological problems.

Chapter 9: Families Of Chidlren With Attention Deficit Disorder

Family Stress

The family of the child with ADD is vulnerable to stress which affects his parents, brothers and sisters. His parents may have previously tried a variety of methods, but many of these proved to be totally ineffective or, at best, of limited value. His behaviour is often unpredictable, and he is less likely to respond to forms of discipline that work for other children. Parents are often baffled by this lack of response and this adds to their frustration. They may be shocked and alarmed by the powerful emotions that he provokes in them.

His brothers and sisters, just like their parents, may not understand his behaviour. They may actually make the situation worse by encouraging or triggering his negative behaviour, either intentionally or by accident.

There is a great deal of ignorance about ADD in the community and parents may listen to unhelpful advice from others, well meaning though it may be. They may devote a great deal of time, effort and money searching for 'cures'. Their stress level is increased further if these methods prove to be ineffective.

The reactions from relatives and friends may generate additional stress. These people may only see him infrequently and usually in a one-to-one situation, and they may not witness the difficulties which his immediate family are forced to cope with. Relatives and friends of the family may not truly understand the daily problems he faces at home and school. They cannot appreciate the many daily frustrations encountered by the child, his parents and teachers.

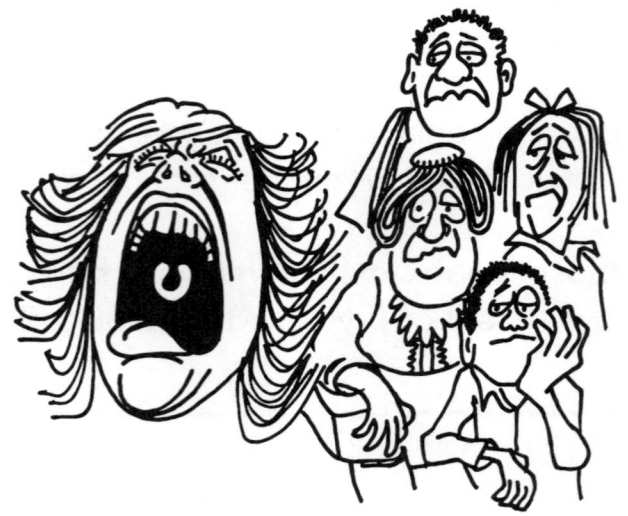

Some parents feel responsible for causing his disability. They feel disappointed when their disciplinary methods do not work, and ultimately they question their own parenting skills. Such powerful emotions may be difficult to eliminate. Their self-esteem often deteriorates. As time goes by, many parents come to feel that they are failures, and they may eventually 'give up' their parenting roles. Other parents may perceive him as a burden and may resent or reject him.

The family may experience many inconveniences, financial costs and lifestyle changes. Outside pressures such as financial problems can impose additional stress on already frustrated parents. His difficulties often impose restrictions on their social and recreational activities.

Living With A Child Who Has ADD

The emotional climate of the household is often greatly influenced by a child with ADD(+H). His unintentional, but erratic and difficult, behaviour may threaten the smooth functioning of his family. His parents need to go through the painful process of accepting that he has a true disability. They often feel disappointed, often experiencing sadness and pain when they realise that he is different from other children. Parents have the task of caring for him on a full-time basis and cannot see any escape from their obligations. This is often much more difficult for single parents.

Some parents find it difficult to live normal lives. They try their best to cope with the very strong and intense emotions triggered by his condition. At the same time they need to develop ways of managing a difficult situation and also their own daily lives.

Parents may find it difficult to enjoy many of the activities they were able to carry out previously. He may be very demanding of the parents' time and energy. Other members of the family, particularly his brothers and sisters, may feel excluded, and this is likely to result in resentment toward him or their parents.

Parents do their best to maintain the wellbeing of everyone in the family. They need expert advice about practical management of his ADD. Many parents benefit from the support of other parents who also have children with ADD.

Chapter 9: Families Of Chidlren With Attention Deficit Disorder

Mothers And Children With ADD

The child with ADD is likely to experience difficulties in carrying out certain tasks, instructions and requests. In most instances his mother is likely to spend more time with him than his father. As a result of this greater contact with him, it is his mother who naturally makes more requests and imposes more instructions on him than his father.

She is likely to respond to his lack of compliance by becoming more forceful, nagging and insistent with him. The constant battles and conflicts, which occur over time, may result in increasing antagonism between them. After a while his mother may ignore the more positive aspects of his behaviour altogether. He may respond to her demands by rejecting his mother's requests and refusing to carry out her instructions and orders.

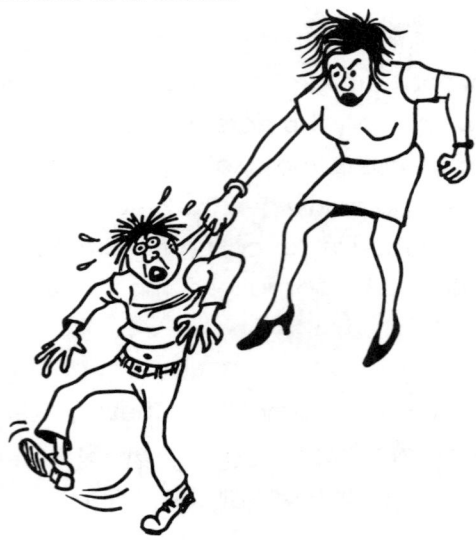

Fathers And Children With ADD

He may experience fewer problems when interacting with his father. There are several possible reasons for this. His father is likely to spend less time with him and therefore he makes fewer requests to comply in carrying out tasks such as schoolwork and chores. Unlike his mother who tends to use reasoning, repetition and affection in gaining his cooperation, his father is possibly less patient and carries out disciplinary measures more readily than his mother.

It is the parent who relies more on reasoning and who devotes more time with him, often his mother, who usually faces more difficulties in gaining cooperation and compliance. The father's larger physical size may intimidate him and this could also be a factor in gaining greater cooperation.

The Relationship Between The Parents

Problems in the relationship between the parents may be aggravated as a result of the differences in the way the child with ADD behaves toward each of them. His father may not believe that there are any great difficulties at home, simply because he does not witness them.

As a result, his father may refuse to admit that the situation is as serious as his mother makes out, and he may blame her for being too sensitive to their son's 'normal enthusiasm'. His father may also believe that she is too permissive or else unwilling to discipline him.

If these differences of opinion between the parents continue, friction between them may well escalate into major disputes and conflict. His mother may feel unsupported and this can lead to further stress for her.

One of the very important principles of managing the child with ADD is the use of consistent methods by both parents. If parents cannot not agree on the most suitable methods of managing their child with ADD, his behaviour may not improve and may even worsen. This adds further pressure on the family.

The Needs Of Other Children In The Family

His temperamental style and poor self-control of behaviour are very frequently misunderstood by his siblings, brothers and sisters alike. His behaviour may be impulsive and aggressive at times, and he may interfere with and spoil many of their games and activities. They may not want to be associated with him and their attitude toward him can be very negative indeed. They are quite likely to become increasingly frustrated and come to resent the effect his demanding behaviour has on their lives.

Chapter 9: Families Of Children With Attention Deficit Disorder

They may respond by rejecting and humiliating him, and this could aggravate his behaviour. The parents are then placed in a very unenviable situation and under immense stress in trying to manage the escalating negative relationships between their children.

Some parents may place extra demands on his siblings because of his lack of compliance. They may expect more of their other children and request that they carry out chores and tasks which his siblings feel are his responsibility. Brothers and sisters often resent these extra demands and accuse the parents of being unfair and favouring him. Siblings may feel neglected by their parents and they resent their brother with ADD(+H) who is constantly demanding of their parents' attention and time. Younger siblings may model or copy his behaviour.

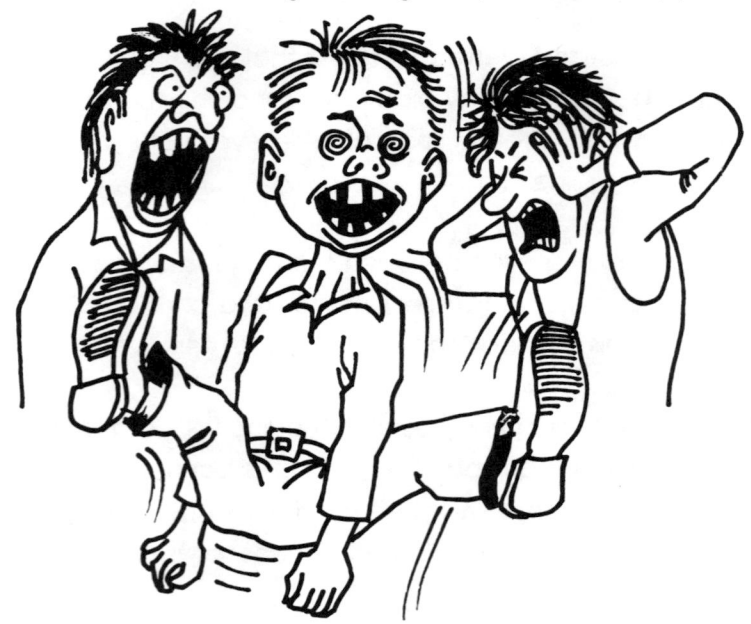

Siblings need to learn skills to help them cope better with his difficult behaviour. Their needs can be easily overlooked. Siblings need to be educated about his ADD so that they are better able to accept him and his disability.

Health Problems Affecting Other Members Of The Family

Various problems that affect other family members, parents and siblings alike, can have major effects on the ways they respond to the child with ADD. These include their emotional and physical health.

Research has shown that the parents of the child with ADD are much more likely to have ADD themselves. There is also a higher incidence of ADD in his brothers and sisters. The parents of the child with ADD are also more likely to suffer from a variety of other disorders including: learning disabilities; antisocial behaviour; drug-related problems, particularly alcoholism; and mood disorders, including depression.

These facts need to be considered in the assessment of the child with ADD. If any of these health problems exist in another member of the family, he or she could benefit greatly by a referral to an appropriate specialist. When the health of other family members is improved, they will be in a much more favourable position to manage the child with ADD in more positive ways.

Reactions Of Families

The child with ADD often has a major impact on his family, particularly if he has ADD(+H). The more severe the condition, the more stress his disability imposes on the family.

Some parents accept that he is experiencing difficulties and they act in positive ways by seeking help as soon as they realise that a problem exists. Others may find it difficult to accept the problem and often experience painful emotions such as guilt and denial for a very long period of time.

Other parents refuse to accept that he is suffering from any difficulty. They may blame other people through sheer frustration and anger. Perhaps a doctor, teacher or school psychologist is the target for this. This blaming, or projection, is their way of coping with a difficult and painful situation. The parents may even blame one another. Patience, time and support are needed to help them face the reality of their circumstances.

Some parents become confused when they receive different suggestions and opinions from a range of well-meaning people. This advice may not be very helpful and it may result in a further delay in the correct diagnosis and treatment. Opinions can emanate from a variety of sources such as friends, relatives, some professionals, television, magazines and newspapers.

His parents are often very anxious and concerned about his future in terms of his schooling, work and career prospects, self-esteem, making friends and being accepted socially.

Parents are often influenced by, and concerned about, the various reactions and opinions of relatives, friends and neighbours. Some are worried about the possibility of having another child with ADD. Others are anxious about losing friends, some of whom have been very supportive to them in the past. Many parents actually withdraw from their social contacts and perhaps from one another. Their isolation serves as a protection from the pain of embarrassment, guilt and shame when facing other people.

Common emotional reactions experienced by parents of the child with ADD include: sadness; disappointment; anger and aggression toward him; feeling inadequate; expecting too much of him; embarrassment; overindulgence; over-protection; self-doubt; poor self-esteem and lack of confidence; and confusion. Such emotional baggage needs to be addressed and dealt with, since it may hamper positive attempts in the management of the child with ADD. His parents may need a great deal of support from someone who truly understands their experience, and this may come from another parent who has a child with ADD or a professional who is well versed in the area.

Eventually most parents accept him as someone who has a disability which can be managed in very positive ways. When they understand that the basis of his difficulties is a result of a developmental and physical problem, they can accept that no one is to blame. They are then able to view him in more positive ways as a person who is special and has needs just like other children.

Some Methods Tried By Parents

Many parents have tried a range of strategies in an attempt to improve his behaviour and performance at home and at school. Although their attempts are well meaning, the strategies used may not be very helpful because they do not appreciate the child's difficulties in self-control of behaviour. Some of the methods are potentially very useful, but they need to be carried out in a proper and consistent manner.

The various methods tried by many parents include: reasoning; tokens and reward systems; compromising; giving him choices; making contracts; setting rules; organising routines; withdrawing privileges; bribery; attending courses in parenting and behaviour management; dietary modification; herbal remedies; criticising; blaming; reprimanding; time out; physical punishment; tranquillisers; tutoring; and the use of coloured lenses.

A Possible Downward Spiral

The use of routine types of discipline are either unsuccessful or only partially effective when applied to the child with ADD(+H). Initially, most parents attempt to deal with his difficult behaviour by trying to ignore it.

When this unacceptable behaviour continues and can no longer be overlooked, they tend to give more frequent orders and demands in an attempt to improve his cooperation. Parents often have to repeat their instructions and requests because he does not carry out the desired behaviour.

Their increasing frustration may result in the issue of progressive threats. If these fail, his parents may resort to physical punishment and other penalties such as loss of privileges or time out.

If their efforts prove to be unsuccessful, his parents may eventually 'give up'. They stop giving commands and let him do as he pleases. They are likely to avoid him and may not supervise him at all. At this stage they often experience feelings of low self-esteem and very little satisfaction in their parenting roles and responsibilities.

An escalation of his difficult behaviour may occur, and this is partly the result of the parents' negative methods and their frustration about the situation. This may result in a condition known as Oppositional Defiant Disorder. If this negative situation continues unabated, then a more serious problem known as Conduct Disorder may develop.

These disorders are described in greater detail in Chapter 15: 'The Future of Children with Attention Deficit Disorder'.

Chapter 9: Families Of Chidlren With Attention Deficit Disorder

Practical Matters

Continuing normal life can be difficult for the family of the child with ADD. Parents often devote a great deal of time and energy in trying to cope with his disability, and at the same time they need to manage their daily lives and those of their other children. Many families do extremely well, but it often takes a great deal of time, effort and energy to perform this balancing act.

ADD is a chronic condition and often poses and imposes various problems on the family. These may include: finding information about ADD and professionals who may help; taking time off work for appointments; coping with their own emotional reactions; determining ways of managing his difficulties; making the necessary adjustments in family life; supporting him at school; supporting other members of the family; and dealing with workers who may be inexperienced in the management of children with ADD and their families.

Single Parent Families

The issue of single parent families is a very important one. Many marriages end in separation or divorce. Research suggests that the divorce rate between the parents of children with ADD is about three times that of the general population. Single parenthood can also result from the death of one of marital partners.

These situations often place a heavy burden on the parent who is left with the responsibility of caring, nurturing and supporting the children. The single parent needs time to cope with intense, sometimes overwhelming, and often ongoing emotional reactions resulting from the loss of the partner and relationship. Over and above this, the single parent needs to support the children in managing and working through similar strong emotions.

Quite apart from these emotional upheavals, the single parent must cope and come to terms with many practical matters. The majority of single parents are mothers. The single mother of a child with ADD may need to manage a very difficult situation on her own, particularly if she has little or no support from her immediate family, other relatives and friends.

Chapter 9: Families Of Chidlren With Attention Deficit Disorder

Her energy level and emotional resources are necessary to meet the needs of her children. These may be quite limited, particularly if she also suffers from an emotional or physical health problem.

The routine activities of organising children for school, laundering, cleaning, shopping, cooking, providing support, helping with schoolwork and getting them ready for bed have to be carried out. There is no escape from these tasks. She may need to keep appointments with doctors, transport him to his tutor, discuss matters with teachers and perform a host of other duties. This can be very difficult particularly if the family is socially or geographically isolated. The child with ADD(+H) can cause major stress for the single parent, particularly when it comes to the mundane and 'boring' activities which simply have to be carried out. There is often no respite for her.

The single parent family is often financially disadvantaged. The parent is often the recipient of welfare payments and these, in most instances, barely cover the essentials. Payment for doctors' services, medication, school and tuition fees may create considerable difficulties. The single parent may not be in a position to provide for the full needs of the child with ADD because the required services are beyond her financial reach. Luxuries are often out of the question, and this can be a great problem for the parent with a demanding and insatiable child who simply wants more and more.

The single parent may not have the time nor energy to socialise with other adults. Obtaining babysitters or respite may prove to be a problem, and she may not be given the opportunity to 'recharge her batteries'. Because she is constantly performing a balancing act for the benefit of the child with ADD and her other children, her own health may suffer.

Separation and divorce may leave children in a crossfire of confusing emotions including anger and blame. They may be placed in the unenviable position of taking sides when one parent undermines what the other parent is trying to achieve in several areas, including the management of the child's disability. Weekend visits with the access parent can prove to be difficult for the custodial parent, particularly if prescribed medication is not given or if other forms of management are not carried out.

Chapter 9: Families Of Children With Attention Deficit Disorder

The access parent, usually the father, may deny that his son suffers from ADD. Alternatively, the child's mother may not provide the father with the necessary information about the child's disability and its proper treatment. As a result, the father may not be in a good position to carry out the necessary and practical methods required to manage the condition.

These real difficulties need to be approached in an effective and consistent manner in order to achieve the best possible outcomes for the child, parents and siblings. Both the parents need to be informed in detail about ADD and its treatment. A clear, practical and flexible plan needs to be devised between the parents and the professionals involved in the child's management.

The single mother needs support from family, friends and relevant community agencies in order to provide her with the important advocacy, educational assistance, counselling and problem solving skills. A good place to start is with an ADD Support Group. It is vital that the single parent maintains her own health so that she can be more effective and better equipped to support her family and, in particular, to manage the ongoing needs of the child with ADD.

Some Final Comments

Most parents are greatly relieved when they find out that the cause for his difficulties has a physical basis, and that it also has a name - Attention Deficit Disorder. Their guilt, anxiety and other emotional reactions are greatly reduced when they are reassured that they are not to blame, and that they have done their best under very difficult circumstances. Once the condition is diagnosed and explained, appropriate treatment may be started. When parents can let go of their emotional baggage, they are in the much more powerful position of accepting practical assessments and treatment for their child's difficulties.

Some parents are disappointed and angry because their child's disability was not diagnosed beforehand, in spite of many consultations with a wide range of professionals. However, the great majority overcome such negative emotions once a correct diagnosis of ADD is made, and particularly when they notice the great improvements and progress he makes when the condition is properly managed.

CHAPTER 10

ASSESSMENT OF CHILDREN WITH ATTENTION DEFICIT DISORDER

Summary

A proper and thorough assessment of the child needs to be carried out before appropriate treatment can be instituted.

Assessment needs to take into account many variables:
- the primary symptoms of ADD
- situational variables
- related conditions
- previously used methods
- family issues

In some situations special psychological or educational assessments may be necessary.

Chapter 10 : Assessment Of Children With Attention Deficit Disorder

The Importance Of Assessment

A thorough and detailed assessment needs to be carried out since the correct diagnosis and proper treatment hinges on it. The process of diagnosing ADD can be very challenging in some situations. ADD is a unique and very individual experience for each child and his family.

It may be a very mild condition in one child whereas another child may suffer from a severe disability to the extent that it creates difficulties in all areas of his life. The possible existence of one or more of the associated conditions, as well as the various complications of ADD also need to be considered. Assessment must take all of these individual differences into account.

The type of assessment which is likely to be carried out depends greatly on the availability, or otherwise, of the resources and expertise in the local community. Some health and psychology professionals have more experience in the area of ADD than others. It is vital that his parents find someone who is experienced in the field of ADD, even though this may prove difficult at times.

The child's total circumstances, including his strengths and weaknesses as well as his home and school situations, need to be fully assessed. The most useful information is obtained from his parents, teachers and the child himself. The use of direct interviews, as well as responses to a range of questionnaires which target specific areas of concern, can also be extremely valuable.

It is useful to view samples of his schoolwork because these may give clues or pointers about the existence of possible learning difficulties. The results of any previous assessments, for example intelligence or other tests, may be useful. But these need to be interpreted with caution because he may not have been under treatment when the testing was carried out. The results may be misleading and not give a true indication of his true capabilities.

Essential Symptoms Of Attention Deficit Disorder

The diagnosis of ADD depends on the continuing presence of a combination of certain symptoms caused by the difficulties he experiences as a result of poor-self-control of behaviour and his temperamental style. In the case of the child with ADD(+H), the difficulties are usually noted as poor selective and sustained attention (often interpreted as 'poor concentration'), poor regulation of general behaviour (often known as 'impulsiveness'), as well as poor control of motor behaviour (often called 'hyperactivity'). The severity of these symptoms vary from one child to another.

The child with ADD(-H) experiences difficulties in focusing his attention and also in sustaining his attention on certain tasks. The criteria used to diagnose ADD(-H) will almost certainly be more refined as the condition becomes more clearly established and defined as the result of ongoing research.

Various behaviour rating scales are often very useful in assessing children with possible ADD and its related conditions. These are easily administered pencil-and-paper tests which are carried out by parents and teachers. They often give useful information and they can support the diagnosis of ADD, particularly when used in conjunction with detailed information obtained from his parents and teachers.

Situational Variability, Associated Conditions And Problems Arising From ADD

Because of the influence of various situations on his self-control, it is vital that information is obtained about those situations and settings which enable him to cope in better ways, and those which are likely to be more troublesome for him.

Parents and teachers often indicate concerns about his academic progress, relationships with other children and other important matters which have a great bearing on his management at home, school and other situations.

The possibility of the existence of related or associated conditions needs to be evaluated. Questions need to be asked about possible problems concerning his self-esteem, bedwetting or soiling, muscle coordination difficulties, specific learning disabilities and Tourette Syndrome. If, after careful questioning, any of these conditions is also suspected, they will need to be properly assessed and managed in their own right.

Chapter 10 : Assessment Of Children With Attention Deficit Disorder

The complications of ADD include poor academic achievement, oppositional defiant disorder, conduct disorder and depression. It is very important that the parents are asked about these because their presence has major implications on subsequent management.

Assessment Of Family Issues

Factors in the child's family can be significant because they may influence the way he is managed on a daily basis. All families are different and their various strengths and weaknesses need to be assessed so that suitable management plans may be arranged to match the specific needs of each child and family.

Some family matters which need to be considered are: family structure; level of understanding of ADD by the parents; the child's understanding of ADD; family functioning and how well family members get on with each other; the effect that his difficulties have on the parents and his brothers and sisters; the quality of the relationship between the child, parents and siblings; the quality of the relationship between the parents; the physical and emotional health of the mother and the father; the possible presence of other children with ADD; and the level of stress in the family.

Assessment Of Previous Management Methods

It is important to determine the parents' ideas about the causes of their child's difficulties and the methods they have previously tried. Answers to questions such as 'who has seen the child in the past and what advice was given ?', 'what methods have been tried ?', 'what worked in the past and what methods work at present ?' and 'what does not work ?' may be very helpful in determining the best type of management for the child and his family.

For example, it may be inadvisable to suggest methods which have previously been proven to be unsuccessful. On the other hand, the parents may not have carried out the strategies in the correct manner, and they may well benefit from advice about applying their methods in more positive ways.

Chapter 10 : Assessment Of Children With Attention Deficit Disorder

Educational Assessment

Other assessments, including various psychological and intelligence tests, may need to be performed. But they do not have to be carried out as a routine. If they are deemed necessary, for example in the case of a child with a possible learning disability, an assessment for this can be arranged after effective treatment for his ADD is instituted with medication. This will enable him to perform relevant assessments and tests under more favourable conditions because of his improved control in both attention and behaviour.

These tests are rather expensive if carried out privately, and such costs need to be taken into account. It is best that they are conducted by a professional who is experienced in dealing with children with the condition. It must be pointed out that most psychological tests may miss the diagnosis of ADD, but they are useful in the assessment of learning and allied problems.

Formal intelligence tests incorporate specific sub-tests which can help analyse his strengths and weaknesses in a range of intellectual and related areas.

Assessments need to consider several important issues concerning the testing of children with ADD. Evidence of ADD is often not noticed in the one-to-one testing situation in which most psychological tests are carried out. It is very well recognised that the behaviour and attention span of the child with ADD can vary greatly in different situations, and he is more likely to experience difficulties in the classroom than in quieter, more interesting, novel and structured settings.

Academic achievement tests can assess a child's specific abilities in reading, writing, spelling and mathematics. Various tests can be used to assess specific aspects of attention, such as the paired associations test, may be carried out before and after medication to determine the effectiveness of drug treatment on attention.

Specific learning disabilities are often diagnosed when there is a significant difference between his intelligence quotient and academic achievement test score in specific areas such as reading, spelling and mathematics.

Chapter 10 : Assessment Of Children With Attention Deficit Disorder

Other Investigations

A medical examination needs to be carried out, although this may sometimes be of little help in diagnosing ADD. Careful observation in the consulting room may alert the doctor to the presence of the child's problems in focusing and sustaining attention, difficulty in controlling muscle activity and the unhappy or stressed facial features of someone who is experiencing poor self-esteem. The doctor may also notice positive and negative interactions between the child and his parents, and also evidence of possible ADD in either of the parents.

The child with ADD is usually very healthy from the physical viewpoint. It is useful to check his height and weight to obtain a baseline so that subsequent growth may be assessed. His hearing and vision should be checked if these have not been carried out previously.

If muscle coordination difficulties are suspected, a more formal assessment by an occupational therapist or physiotherapist may be indicated. This should be preferably carried out after treatment of his ADD has been started.

Special neuro-electrical tests measure the electrical activity in various parts of the brain. These investigations include computerised electroencephalography (EEG) and related brain mapping techniques which may demonstrate atypical electrical activity in immature areas of the brain. These tests may be of use in the assessment of learning disabilities. Related tests such as auditory-evoked and visually-evoked responses, may also show up the immaturity in the transmission of the electrical nerve impulses in certain parts of the brain. These investigations are available in some centres.

Some newer tests are currently the subject of research. For example positron emission tomography (PET) is showing great promise as a research tool, but the equipment is extremely expensive and not readily available. PET has demonstrated reduced blood flow and reduced sugar uptake in the areas of the brain involved in the control and regulation of behaviour in people with ADD.

ADD can usually be diagnosed on the basis of information derived from parent and teacher interviews and these specialised tests are usually unnecessary.

Chapter 10 : Assessment Of Children With Attention Deficit Disorder

Final Comments

Assessment needs to take into account a variety of many different but related factors. These all need to be considered carefully so that a practical diagnosis may be made as a prelude to planning a total approach to the management of the child within his family. The assessment process needs to be broadly based, and take into account the many factors which are likely to impinge on management. The specific assessments should be aimed at addressing the individual needs of the child and his family. The important first step is to confirm or refute the diagnosis of ADD.

Because ADD is a condition which can be quite variable, various modifications to treatment may be needed from time to time. Assessment is not a static issue and must be carried out on a repeated basis because of the changing circumstances and needs of the child and his family.

Some of the important matters concerning the assessment of the child with possible ADD are outlined in Appendix 2: 'Assessment - Issues For Parents' and also in Appendix 3: 'Assessment - Teacher Issues'.

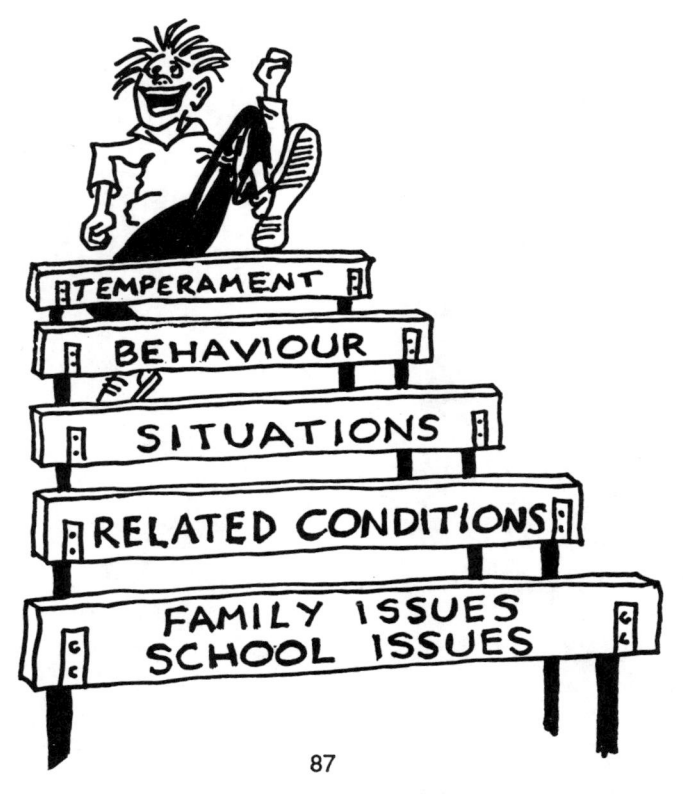

CHAPTER 11

GENERAL ASPECTS OF MANAGEMENT

> ### Summary
>
> Management is a continuous process and it should consider the unique needs of each child and family.
>
> Effective treatments include various combinations of medical, psychological and educational strategies.
>
> A team effort is required and this necessarily involves the child with ADD, his family, teachers and other professionals.
>
> All members of the team need to communicate and work closely together.

Chapter 11 : General Aspects Of Management

Critical Issues Involved In Management

ADD cannot be cured, but it can usually be well controlled. Gaining control is important in order to enable him to function better in various aspects of his daily life at home, school and socially. Self-control is needed to prevent many of the potential difficulties he is likely to face. It is also important to prevent some of the potential major emotional, social, career and other problems in his later life.

The main goal of management is to enable the child with ADD to function in the best possible way in spite of his disability. In other words, management involves the use of the best available means to 'normalise' his attention and behaviour control so that he is more able to achieve his full potential in the full range of activities.

Management needs to be directed at improving the electrical and chemical function of the brain, which usually involves the use of medication, as well as a variety of other methods when necessary. These are aimed at modifying the situations which may have a negative influence on his self-control of behaviour and attention.

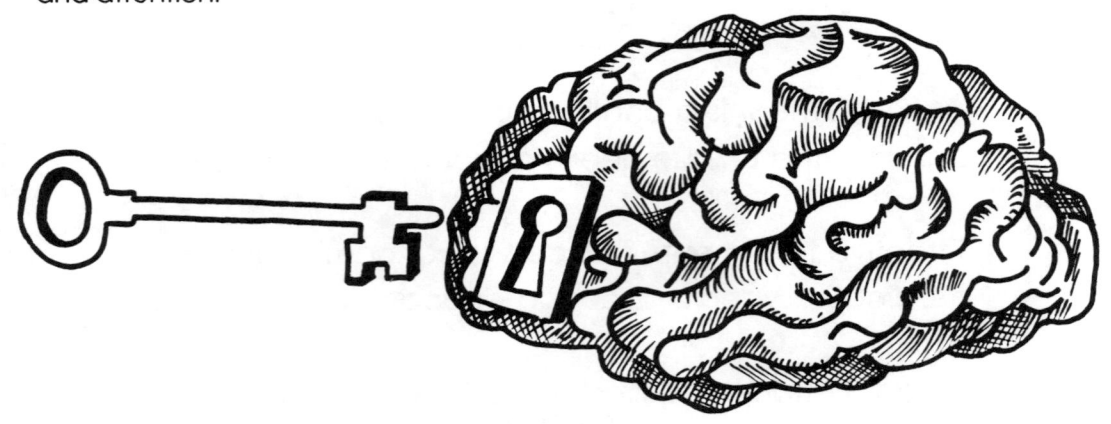

Because of the variable nature of ADD, management involves a continuous process of awareness, regular assessment of his condition and of his progress, and modifying specific treatments when necessary. Management needs to be carried out in the context of his family, school and other situations. Each child with ADD is unique and so is his situation. The various treatments used must suit his individual needs and those of his family. A range of treatments may be needed, depending on the various factors determined in the assessment.

Chapter 11 : General Aspects Of Management

Searching For Help

Finding the 'right' professional to assist the child and his family can be a major problem for many parents. Such experts may be few and far between, and his parents may search for many months, or even years, before finding someone who understands their situation.

Many parents are very confused about their child's behaviour and problems in school work and they often 'shop around' in an attempt to find someone who can help. They may begin their search in various different places. For instance friends, teachers, the family doctor or a psychologist may suggest a referral to someone who specialises in the area of ADD. His parents may be lucky and meet another parent who has a child with ADD receiving suitable management.

Advice may be sought through a local ADD Support Group and the parents are often reassured to discover that they are not alone. Parents are usually greatly relieved when they find someone who understands their personal predicament and who can empathise with them.

The specialist must be able to communicate well with both the child and his parents. They want clear and accurate information about ADD. Parents often want to know about causes for his various difficulties as well as his prospects for the future. They need straightforward information about the type of assessment required, the aims of treatment, details about the available treatments, and the costs involved.

The parents and child must be given the opportunity to ask questions and clarify various matters which are of concern to them. They must not be blamed for causing or being responsible for the child's difficulties.

A Team Approach

The main members of the management team are the child himself, the parents and his teachers. They need to work closely together at all times. Assessment of his progress in the areas of behaviour, learning, self-esteem and socialisation should be carried out on a regular basis.

Chapter 11 : General Aspects Of Management

They also need to review their strategies and determine which ones are working well and which ones are no longer helpful. If necessary they may need to alter or modify their approaches according to the needs of the child. The members of the team should carry out their activities in a consistent way so that everyone is clear about what is being done and what needs to be done.

The team needs information and appropriate 'training' in the management of the child with ADD. This may be difficult, particularly for the busy teacher. Other members of the child's family, for example older brothers or sisters, can benefit greatly in learning about his ADD and so enable them to understand why he is experiencing his various difficulties. This increased awareness will enable them to become useful members of the management team.

Other members of the team may be a paediatrician and a psychologist. These consultants can be very helpful in carrying out regular assessments, discussing various parental concerns, and also modifying management when necessary. As ADD is frequently a variable condition, and because family situations may alter from time to time, regular follow-up and review are important. A number of families need a great deal of support. Telephone contact with these people should be encouraged in cases where there is an unexpected crisis at home or at school, and in case treatment needs to be changed suddenly.

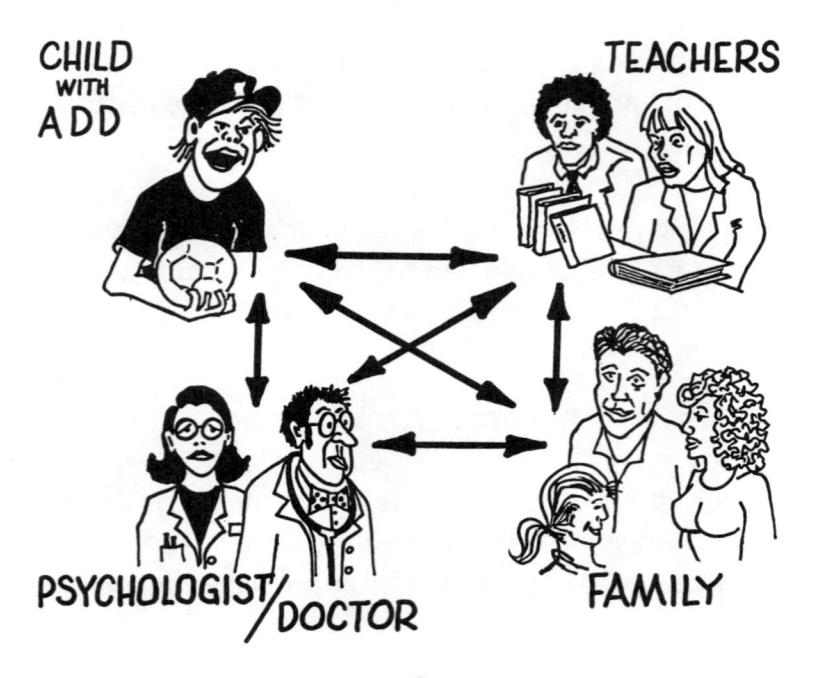

Chapter 11 : General Aspects Of Management

Other professionals may also need to be involved at some stage, depending on the presence, or otherwise, of any related conditions. They may include: a speech pathologist for management of language and articulation disorders; a remedial or special education teacher to help the child who experiences learning difficulties; a physiotherapist or occupational therapist to help the child with muscle coordination difficulties; a school psychologist who may carry out intellectual and academic assessments, and who may also suggest various practical classroom interventions.

Treatments That Don't Work

A range of different treatment methods have been tried in the past as attempts to manage children with ADD. Some methods have been proven to be useful whereas others are of little, if any, value.

Methods which have been shown to be ineffective are: dietary treatments, including the elimination of certain food colourings, natural salicylates, sugars and a variety of additives; chiropractic treatment; hypnotherapy; megavitamin therapy (high doses of vitamins); long-term psychotherapy (talking therapy); and sensory integration therapy. None of these can be recommended. These ineffective treatments may be quite expensive and time consuming to carry out. Yet there are some people, including well-meaning friends, relatives and various professionals, who still recommend their use.

Because there are many desperate parents who are willing to try anything to help their children, they may listen to those people whose advice is unhelpful. Parents may be convinced to try one or more of these unproven or disproven methods. Unfortunately this delays the introduction and use of more suitable and effective treatments, and may add to the existing frustration at home.

Effective Treatments

There are three main broad groups of effective treatments available. These involve various medical, psychological and educational methods. Each will be discussed in detail in the next three chapters. Children who suffer from the more

Chapter 11 : General Aspects Of Management

severe forms of ADD often require a combination of interventions. Each child with ADD is unique. The types of treatment required depend very much on a number of factors which have been described in previous chapters. Some of these factors include: the severity of his ADD; the presence, or otherwise, of associated conditions or complications; and various family matters.

The more 'complicated' the situation, the more 'complex' the management is likely to be. Some children with mild ADD may require medication only. The child with multiple difficulties may need medication, educational interventions and a range of psychological methods. These methods often enhance each other, and this relationship is illustrated in the figure shown below.

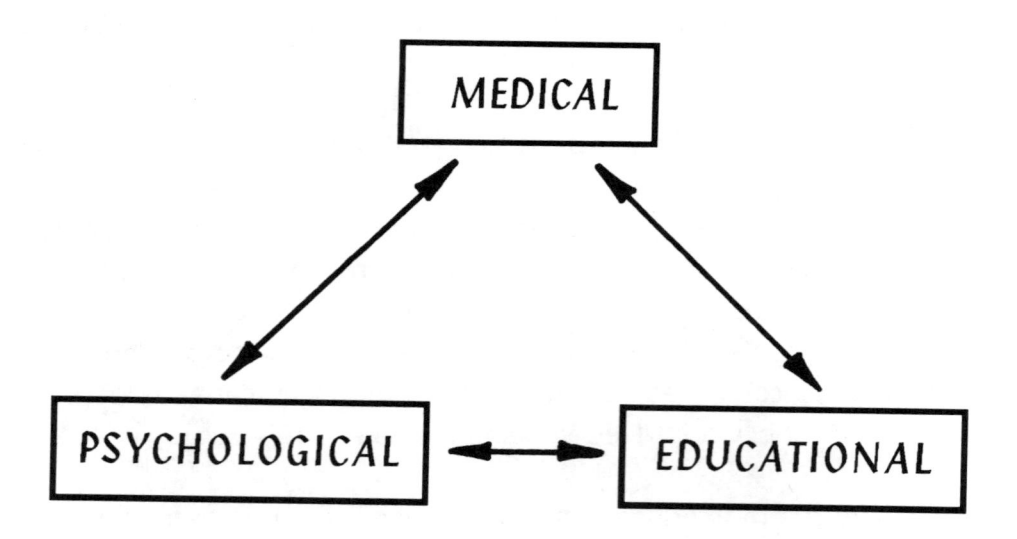

CHAPTER 12

MEDICAL TREATMENT

> **Summary**
>
> Medication has been shown to be the single most valuable form of treatment for ADD.
>
> The aim of medication treatment is to enable the child to increase his self-control by 'correcting' the function of a part of the brain which is operating in an inefficient way.
>
> The challenge is to determine the most appropriate medication, using the smallest effective dose and with the fewest side-effects, and to suit the needs of the child and his family.

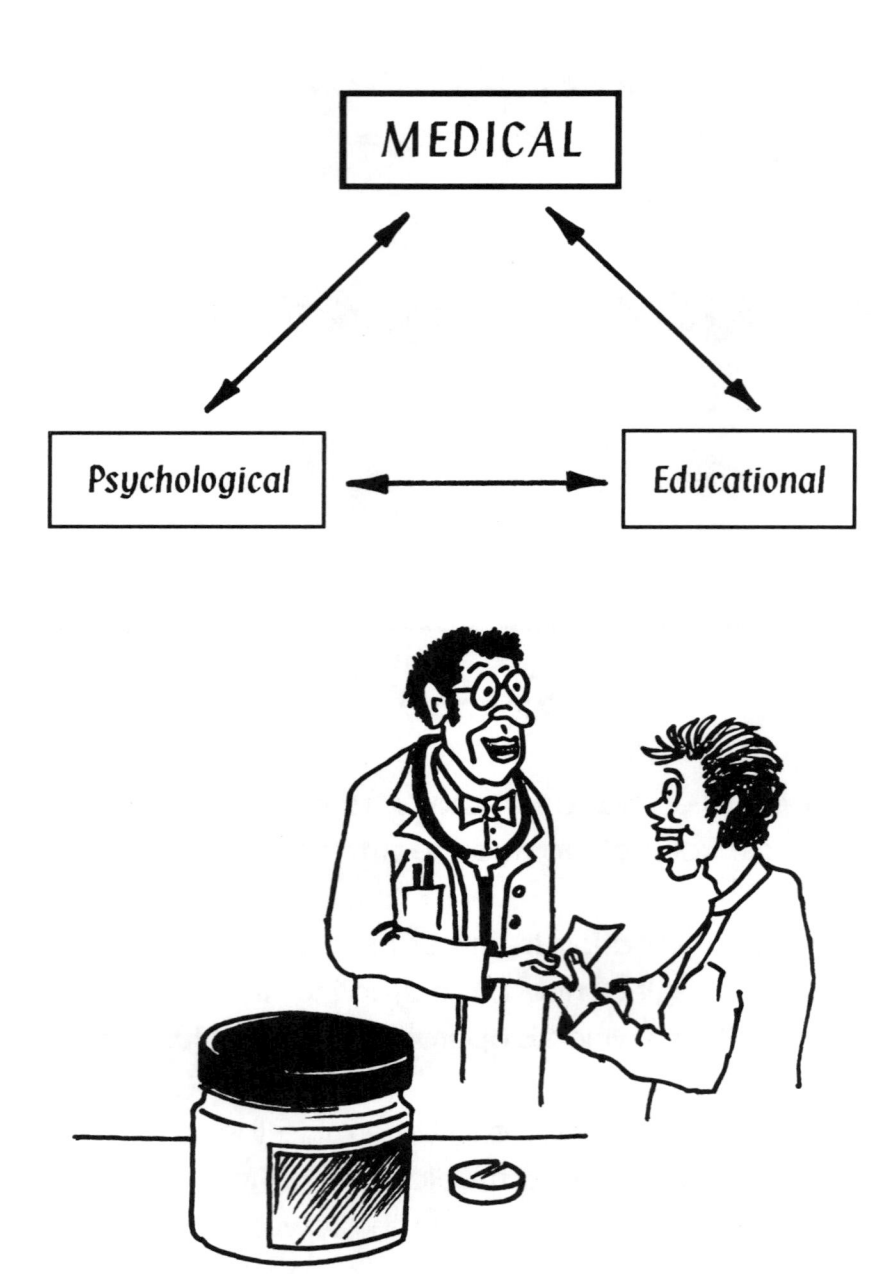

Chapter 12 : Medical Treatment

Chapter 12 : Medical Treatment

Why Medication ?

The symptoms of ADD result from the inefficient and immature function of a part of the brain. This results in poor availability of important chemical messengers, or neurotransmitters, which send messages from one nerve cell to another. It is this abnormality which is thought to be corrected by stimulant medication. They 'switch on' or 'stimulate' the inefficiently operating chemical/electrical system so that it can work in a more normal and effective way.

Hundreds of studies have repeatedly shown that medication is extremely useful in treating ADD, far more so than any other single form of treatment. This type of intervention is all that is needed in many cases, especially in children who have mild ADD without complications.

The response to the 'right' medication is often dramatic and rapid. Because medication deals with the fundamental problem, it optimises the use of other forms of treatment if they are necessary. In other words, after 'correcting' the child's internal environment, appropriate 'external' strategies are more likely to be effective when used in conjunction with medication.

Types Of Medication

The most commonly used medications used in the treatment of ADD are known as the stimulants. Those currently available in Australia are dexamphetamine and methylphenidate (Ritalin). They are effective in the majority of children with ADD. Their effect is often noticed within one hour of taking the correct dose, and they may need to be taken 3 or 4 times a day because of their short action of about 4 hours.

Other medications may need to be used if the child's ADD is not controlled by the stimulants, or if they produce troublesome side-effects. These alternatives include: imipramine, desipramine, moclobemide and fluoxetine, all of which are also used for the treatment of depression. They may be very effective in controlling the symptoms of ADD in some children.

Chapter 12 : Medical Treatment

Clonidine has been shown to be effective in enabling many children to control their impulsive, hyperactive and aggressive behaviour. It may be added to the stimulants, and together they can bring about considerable improvements in his behaviour. (Sometimes thioridazine is used for behavioural control).

Taking Control

Once the medication begins to act, the child is able to take increasing control of his behaviour and is more able to focus and sustain his attention in a far more regular and consistent way. His parents, siblings and teachers often alter their previous negative ways of viewing and managing him. They then begin to take more notice of his positive qualities which were previously hidden behind his disability. They are able to approach and manage him in more constructive ways. The stress levels of the child, family and teachers decline greatly and this often results in great benefits for everyone concerned.

Side-Effects Of The Stimulants

All drugs have their side-effects and this applies also to the stimulants. Some children do not experience any side-effects, and those who do usually suffer temporary problems which are of nuisance value only. The stimulants are not addictive and they do not produce growth difficulties nor other long-term side-effects at the dosages used to treat ADD.

The commonest short-term side-effects are crying, headaches, abdominal pain and irritability which last for a very few days only. They may also produce a reduction in his appetite and difficulty in getting to sleep. Such side-effects may persist for several days or perhaps several weeks. Some children experience 'rebound', or a deterioration in behaviour when the effects of the medication wear off. Rebound can usually be managed by altering the dosage of the medication.

Less common are drowsiness and a reduction in muscle activity, both of which indicate that the dosage is too high and needs to be reduced. A relatively rare complication is the development of involuntary movements or tics, and this may require a reduction in the dose or a change in medication.

Chapter 12 : Medical Treatment

Some children develop a tolerance or resistance to stimulant medication. This is noticed when the symptoms of his ADD return after months or even years of successful treatment. Tolerance is usually temporary but it does necessitate a change of medication for a while, and the previously effective medication can be reintroduced later when it is likely to be effective once again.

Combinations Of Medications

The stimulant medications are often effective in controlling all symptoms of the disability, including his difficulties in regulating his behaviour and attention. In some cases, however, a combination of medications is needed. The types of medication required depend on the specific target symptoms and behaviours which need to be managed.

For example, if his difficulties in paying attention dramatically improve with the use of stimulant medication but his aggressive or impulsive behaviour continue to be a concern, the addition of clonidine often results in marked improvement in his ability to control his behaviour.

If he continues to appear depressed or his poor self-esteem continues to be a concern whilst taking stimulants, his mood may lift significantly with the addition of one of the antidepressants, including imipramine or moclobemide. These may have the additional benefit of helping him control other symptoms of ADD.

He may have bedwetting as a related condition. Imipramine has been shown to be of great value in managing this frustrating condition and it may be added to the stimulants.

Many children with Tourette Syndrome have ADD as well. The tics or involuntary movements of Tourette Syndrome may be helped significantly with clonidine or other medications. His ADD, however, needs to be treated in its own right. Care needs to be taken in this situation because the stimulants may aggravate the involuntary movements of Tourette Syndrome. If these tics become apparent, they can usually be very easily controlled with the use of various medications, including clonidine.

Chapter 12 : Medical Treatment

What Medications Don't Do

The use of medication simply allows the child to take increasing control of his ADD and improves the likelihood of his full potential to be reached. They are not 'smart drugs' and they do not increase his intelligence, but they enable him to pay increasing attention and perform better in various academic subjects. The improvement in attention makes it easier for him to 'catch up' in those subjects in which he is underachieving. Medications do not 'cure' specific learning disabilities, although they can significantly enhance the effectiveness of special education methods.

Medication will not transform him into a perfectly behaved child overnight. All children have their good and bad days, but the child with untreated ADD(+H) is more likely to have 'bad' days than other children. Medication enables him to improve the control he has over his behaviour, but he is still prone to be influenced by various situational factors. In other words, he may continue to be vulnerable to the ups and downs of daily living, just like anyone else. In other words, medication will not cure nor prevent all behavioural 'hiccups'.

Monitoring Of Medication

ADD is a chronic disability and the symptoms are quite variable. Regular review is important. It is crucial to determine progress and to modify treatment if this is necessary. Alterations to the type of medication and dosage may be needed from time to time. Height and weight need to be checked periodically to ensure that his growth is progressing in a satisfactory way.

Community Attitudes About Medication

The use of medications for the management of ADD is frowned upon by many people. Some have strong attitudes about the use of drugs for any condition, let alone their use in treating the child with ADD. The truth of the matter is that the use of stimulant medication in ADD is based on strong scientific evidence, and it has been shown to positively influence the lives of many children and with no long-term side effects.

Chapter 12 : Medical Treatment

It is an unfortunate fact that some people do not understand the nature of ADD, its cause and how medications work in the management of this condition. This lack of insight can be be detrimental to the child with ADD and his family. Those people who refuse to accept that medications have any role in the treatment of ADD may influence and convince parents to avoid their use and so deprive the child of a very useful form of treatment.

Others consider that medications should be used only as a last resort. But it could be argued that medications should be the first line of treatment, since they have been proven scientifically to be effective. Medications work quickly, often producing a dramatic improvement in his self-control and various other symptoms of ADD. They are extremely simple to use and are far less time- and energy-consuming than other strategies. Many of the medications used are inexpensive and they enhance other forms of treatment.

Some Final Comments

Many children with ADD cannot function properly without the use of medication. The correct dose and timing of administration of medication may need to be modified from time to time.

The aim of treatment with medication is to achieve the best possible response with the fewest possible side effects at the smallest possible dose and the least financial cost. Many children with mild symptoms often do exceptionally well with medication alone, and they may not require any other type of intervention.

Some of the other medications may be given a trial if the stimulants prove to be ineffective. The timing of medication needs to be adjusted to suit the needs of the child at home and at school. Because of the short action of the stimulants, they need to be taken at school and this requires cooperation between the family and school staff. Schools should incorporate specific plans to serve the needs of the child to take medication at specified times.

Teenagers and older children with ADD need to discuss all aspects of their ADD, including treatment with medication. They should clarify any issues about the use of medication with their doctor

Chapter 12 : Medical Treatment

Some doctors suggest 'drug holidays' and recommend that the child with ADD does not take medication after school, on weekends, or during vacations. This may be appropriate for the child with ADD(-H) who does not need to perform activities requiring sustained attention at these times. However, the disability of ADD does not 'switch off' during these times, and the child with severe ADD(+H) usually needs to take medication every day to enable him to improve his self-control. It is vital that a flexible plan regarding the administration of medication be devised in conjunction with the doctor.

Some parents have difficulty in accepting the use of long-term medication by their child. This issue needs to be handled sensitively. These parents need time to contemplate the benefits and side-effects of the various forms of treatment, and perhaps speak to other parents who have a child with ADD who is taking medication. It is the doctor's duty to provide parents with accurate information about medication and other forms of treatment for ADD so that they are in a better position to make informed decisions about their child's management.

Many of the symptoms of ADD may improve and some may disappear by the late teenage years in many children. Medication is used as a holding strategy while awaiting the prospect that further maturation of the brain will take place so that hopefully he will 'outgrow' his ADD. It is impossible to predict whether or not this will happen in any individual child. The child who 'outgrows' his condition does not need to continue to take his medication. Others who are less fortunate may need to continue taking medication indefinitely.

The possible positive effects of medication are summarised in Appendix 4: 'The Benefits Of Medication'.

CHAPTER 13

PSYCHOLOGICAL MANAGEMENT

> **Summary**
>
> Specific psychological strategies, particularly behavioural methods, can be very useful in helping the child with ADD take control.
>
> Modifications to his environment may be made in a variety of situations and these enable him to improve his self-control.
>
> The proper use of psychological methods requires an understanding of certain concepts and the strict adherence to carefully designed plans and procedures.

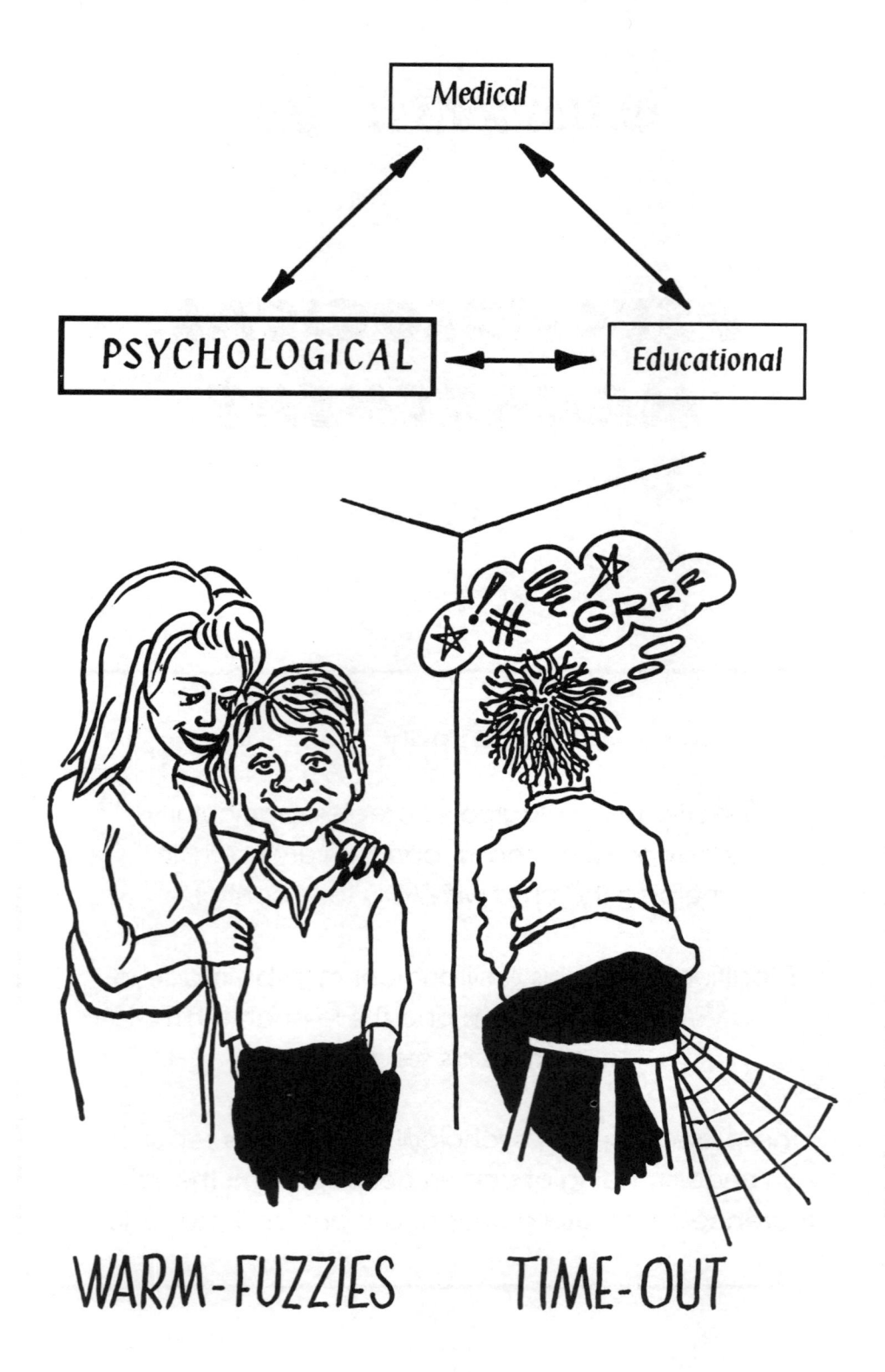

Chapter 13 : Psychological Management

WARM-FUZZIES   TIME-OUT

Chapter 13 : Psychological Management

Why Psychological Methods ?

The child's self-control often improves greatly with the use of medication and he is better able to control his behaviour. The quality of his life often improves dramatically. Other people including his parents, siblings, teachers and peers respond to him in more positive ways. However, medications may not alleviate all of his symptoms.

Some parents have various concerns about the long-term use of medication by their child and may not want him to take this form of treatment. There may be several reasons for this, and their wishes need to be respected. However, they need to have the necessary and accurate information about medication so that they may make an informed decision.

For these and other reasons, some of the alternative methods of treatment may need to be considered. But before any method is instituted, the parents need to understand their child's condition and the reasons he experiences the many difficulties he encounters. As already pointed out, these include his problems in controlling attention and behaviour particularly in response to instructions,and this is more of a problem when other stimuli compete with their requests.

Strategies used for the child with ADD should concentrate on the prevention of those situations which are likely to create problems for him. They also need to focus on actively dealing with various behaviour difficulties when they occur. Psychological strategies can be useful in both these areas.

Parent Counselling And Education

The child's parents must understand all aspects of his condition, how it affects him and the reasons for his poor self-control and self-motivation.

He is likely to experience more difficulties than other children in carrying out certain tasks and behaviours. The adults in his life need to remember that he is less responsive to the usual methods of behaviour management that work for other children. This makes it more probable that his parents and teachers will experience some difficulties and frustrations in their interactions with him.

Chapter 13 : Psychological Management

Common Behaviour Problems

Because of his difficulties in self-control, the child with ADD may exhibit a variety of behaviours which tend to occur time and time again. Some of the specific behaviours that his parents may complain of include: lying and stealing; temper tantrums; swearing; answering back and being argumentative; teasing others; ignoring requests or refusing to carry out requests or instructions; destroying property; fighting with others; fidgeting; excessive talking, yelling or screaming; and disrupting the activities of others.

These same behaviours may also occur at school. In addition, he may have problems with activities involved in learning. For example he may experience problems in: producing neat work; getting organised; starting tasks; maintaining on-task behaviour; and completing schoolwork, assignments and projects.

It is highly desirable that his parents and teachers identify and target the specific troublesome behaviours he exhibits before instituting any plans and programs to help him overcome them.

Important Points About Using Psychological Methods

Parents and teachers need to grasp some of the important concepts involved in the use of the various psychological methods. If these are not followed, there is a likelihood that potentially effective methods will not work in the desired way.

All children, but particularly those with ADD, respond better to praise, positive feedback or rewards than to punishment. In the case of the child with ADD, such rewards need to be given frequently in order for them to be effective. The use of these positive methods and rewarding acceptable behaviour increases the likelihood of such behaviour being repeated in the future. These rewards must be sufficiently powerful and important to him in order to act as incentives or motivational tools. They need to be given frequently.

He may need to be disciplined from time to time, but reprimands on their own are unlikely to alter his behaviour. If they are to be used at all, negative means must be combined with rewards when he exhibits acceptable behaviour.

Chapter 13 : Psychological Management

The specific situations which trigger or promote his unacceptable behaviour should be identified. Specific behaviours need to be targeted. That is, parents and teachers need to be clear about what they expect him to do, rather than concentrate solely on what he is not meant to do. Their expectations need to be explained and repeated frequently and they must not make the assumption that he automatically knows what is expected of him.

Specific programs and procedures aimed at managing his behaviour need to be planned and followed very carefully. All consequences, including rewards and reprimands, need to be dispensed immediately after he carries out the behaviour in question.

Parents may unintentionally increase the likelihood of his undesirable behaviour being carried out again if they avoid disciplining or reprimanding him when such measures are necessary and indicated. He may surmise, 'I got away with it this time, so I'll try it again. Hopefully I'll get away with it next time as well.'

Both his parents need to be consistent in the way they deal with his behaviour. They must cooperate with each other and back up each other's efforts. This reduces the possibility of successful use of 'divide and conquer' tactics by the child. Otherwise he may end up controlling his parents.

He should not be punished for behaviours directly caused by his ADD and over which he has little control. This includes his difficulties in paying attention and forgetfulness.

Modifications may need to be made in any program from time to time. These depend on a number of factors such as the physical space and layout of the home, the health of the parents, the age and number of children living at home and other family matters.

Some Important Hints

Parents and teachers need to continually remind themselves about important factors which influence his behaviour. His ADD provides a challenge for these adults in the ways they manage him at home and at school. They must accept

Chapter 13 : Psychological Management

that he has a disability which results in difficulties with self-control. The child with ADD is not a 'problem child' but rather a 'child who has a problem'. It must be realised that there is no cure for ADD, and that the whole point of management is to allow him to function as normally as possible in spite of his disability.

Behaviour management is one aspect of total treatment and it has limitations, just like the other treatments. Parents and teachers must refrain from blaming themselves for his difficulties in controlling behaviour. They need to accept that the management road is often a rocky one, with many ups and downs, many good days and some bad days.

Parents must learn to accept that they cannot be perfect all the time. They need time and patience to acquire and practise some special skills. These are fundamental elements necessary to manage the child with ADD.

Parents need to manage their own health problems and the various stresses in their own lives. Such stresses may aggravate his behaviour. By managing their own health problems they will be in a better position to deal with his situation in more effective ways.

Without realising it, adults may contribute to his problems with behaviour. They need to be aware of both the useful and unhelpful methods they are currently using, and either change or modify them if necessary. Some of the methods that are unlikely to work include: yelling and screaming; physical punishment; focusing only on his problem behaviours and ignoring his positive ones; not carrying out previously agreed upon consequences; and repeating instructions too often.

Planning - The Key To Prevention

Parents and teachers may become frustrated by his repeated unacceptable behaviour which may escalate and get out of control from time to time. It is often far better and easier to try to prevent such outbursts than to deal with them once this happens. Unfortunately they may have developed some ineffective approaches over a long period of time. They need to learn more effective skills while 'unlearning' less successful methods.

Chapter 13 : Psychological Management

Careful planning, anticipation and monitoring of his behaviour are quite critical in preventing episodes of difficult behaviour. Before such planning takes place it is vital that everyone involved in his management understands how he 'ticks' and under which conditions and situations he is likely to experience difficulties.

Some of the important requirements in preventing his unacceptable behaviour from occurring in the first place, and managing them when they actually occur include: parents and teachers working together as a team and in a consistent way; ensuring him of a supportive and safe family environment; demonstrating affection and approval during the good times; and ensuring that he knows he is accepted, and that he is a valued member of the family, in spite of his disability.

The planning of specific strategies depends on certain crucial psychological concepts. These must take into account the difficulties he experiences as a result of the problems he has in regulating his behaviour.

The important principles include:

- Identifying specific target behaviours.

- Identifying and monitoring those situations and incidents which trigger his unacceptable behaviours.

- Determining ways of preventing these incidents from happening. For example, if his behaviour is a problem when his parents are talking on the telephone, they may arrange to make their calls while he is attending school and also encourage their friends to call at these times.

- Maintaining close and regular contact with his teachers and checking his behaviour at school. His parents and teachers need to carry out programs which are consistent across both home and school settings. A consistent approach is fundamental in the managing the child with ADD.

- Developing a regular routine and pattern for daily activities, for example meal times, bathing, homework, watching television and going to bed.

- Avoiding put-downs and negative labels about his temperament or personality, and other qualities over which he has little control.

Chapter 13 : Psychological Management

- Ignoring minor behaviour infringements if possible. Parents and teachers run the risk of an escalation in his behaviour if they make a big issue of minor irritating behaviour.

- Modifying the home and class environment so that they are safe. Avoiding 'overstimulation' so that the number of stimuli in his immediate environment are suitable for his needs, and which are unlikely to trigger poor self-control.

- Rewarding acceptable behaviour immediately after it occurs, using praise and other positive methods.

- Arranging physically active exercise on a regular basis.

- Discussing his feelings regularly and trying to understand important issues from his point of view.

- Providing him with tasks and activities which he can complete within a short time frame.

- Allowing him to work at his own pace within reasonable time limits.

- Giving him brief and exact directions and instructions, but only when his total undivided attention is obtained. It is important to block out other distractions when giving instructions. Requests may need to be repeated several times.

- Increasing his awareness of how his behaviour affects others.

- Providing him with suggestions for alternative behaviour, and not expecting him to automatically know what is required of him. The words 'don't' and 'stop' do not provide him with the tools and information about what he is required to do as a substitute for unacceptable behaviour.

- Giving him immediate feedback for acceptable behaviour.

- Arranging opportunities for him to interact with one or two other children at a time, and avoiding his involvement in large groups.

- Giving him one-to-one attention on a regular basis.

These suggestions are easy to put down on paper, but they may take considerable time and effort to put into practice. It is best to start with one or two of those methods with which his parents and teachers feel comfortable and which are most likely to meet with some success.

Once this is achieved, other methods may be introduced. It is more likely that he will experience increasing achievement over his situation because these preventive strategies will enable him to increase his self-control. The adults in his life need to provide him with the necessary and valuable tools which enable him to function in more positive ways.

There are some special psychological techniques which have been proven to be effective when applied to children with ADD. Some of these strategies are outlined in Appendix 5: 'Some Specific Psychological Strategies'.

Management Of Situational Variables

The child with ADD is greatly influenced by the prevailing situations in which he finds himself. It is usually possible to plan ahead, organise and arrange these different settings so that they work to his advantage.

The following suggestions may prompt parents and teachers to consider the types of situational changes which could improve his behaviour and attention. Adults may: arrange his environment so that it is more colourful and stimulating; increase the amount of one-to-one contact with him; encourage him to use computers; encourage him to spend more time on his own; avoid placing unnecessary demands on him; give immediate rewards for positive behaviour and also for completion of assigned tasks; arrange more difficult tasks to be carried out in the morning and early afternoon.

These strategies may involve adding items to his environment, and so make this more stimulating. In other instances certain things may be removed from his environment, thereby reducing any unnecessary distractions and improving his ability to focus and sustain his attention.

Alternatively, his environment may be better organised with the use of a diary, notebook or notice board so that he is more easily reminded of important and relevant messages, timetables and other matters.

Chapter 13 : Psychological Management

Some situations are better avoided. For instance, parents may need to make their phone calls, do their shopping or visit their friends when he is at school.

Other Strategies

The child with ADD may have difficulties in a range of personal skills. These skills may need to be learned in special programs, and they are best carried out in conjunction with the use of medication. The kinds of skills to be learned depend on the types of difficulties he is experiencing. Some areas in which additional help may be of value include: problem solving; planning and organisational skills; study and work skills; time management; improving self-esteem; improving self-control, including control of anger; relaxation and stress management skills; and communication skills and team working.

The scope of this book does not allow these to be discussed here. Some of the essential issues involved in the development of these skills are summarised in Appendix 6: 'Skills Development'. If parents wish to pursue these matters, they should consult with relevant private specialists or community agencies in their local area.

Psychological Help For The Family

Stress in the family can be a significant problem. There is also an increased likelihood of psychological problems affecting the parents. They may need to seek assistance to help them cope and improve family functioning. Once their own quality of life improves, they will be in a better position to help the child with ADD and their other children. For example, if depression is a significant problem for a parent, it is often very worthwhile that a psychiatric assessment be sought so that suitable treatment may be instituted.

Sometimes family therapy is indicated. The intention of this is to improve family interactions and communication between all members of the family. Parents may learn more positive ways of relating to the child with ADD. Family therapy may be useful in a range of other areas such as improving parenting skills, learning effective forms of child management, improving the marital relationship, relieving family stress, resolving guilt and other negative emotional reactions.

Chapter 13 : Psychological Management

Oppositional And Aggressive Behaviour

The child with ADD(+H) often displays oppositional and sometimes aggressive behaviour. These behaviours may be difficult to manage. Physical punishment is of little value because it often results in escalating anger in both the child and his parents. This often leads to blaming and put-downs, resentment and rage, as well as verbal and physical retaliation by the child.

These confrontations do not bring about the intended result, and he does not necessarily reflect or think about what he has done. His behaviour is unlikely to change. Physical punishment should be avoided at all costs, and this may take considerable constraint on the part of the parents. They may need to learn alternative positive skills such as the time out procedure which is described in Appendix 5: 'Some Specific Psychological Strategies'.

Parents frequently use the words 'no', 'don't' and 'stop', but these are almost foreign to the child with ADD(+H). When parents use them, he may be triggered into a temper tantrum or rage attack.

Alternatively he may confront them with a barrage of 'why ?' or 'why can't I ?' questions and this is likely to provoke the parents into repeating their negative statement or else give reasons for it.

Before they know it, they are drawn into an escalating to-and-fro interchange of negative reactions. Parents must learn to use these words once only, and if the instruction is not obeyed, they need to quickly carry out a previously planned and agreed upon consequence. Once again, the time out procedure may be of value.

It is very easy for parents to get caught up in a vicious spiral of angry verbal exchanges with the child who is defiant, oppositional or angry. They must avoid being drawn into arguments and must refuse all attempts at explaining and reasoning. Parents must hold their ground and remain silent. There can be no fight if the parents opt out, since a fight needs at least two opponents. Parents must realise that he may exaggerate his verbal abuse, but they must refrain from giving in to his hostility and aggression.

Chapter 13 : Psychological Management

For the child with ADD(+H), temper tantrums may be an habitual way of reacting to the slightest provocation. During such tantrums he may become totally out of control. Parents need to realise that he is beyond reach and reasoning when he is in the midst of a blind rage.

It is vital that they avoid being drawn into any encounter with him and to avoid taking anything he says in a personal way. He simply needs time to settle down, and this may take several minutes or even hours.

Some Final Comments

Psychological interventions need to be individualised to fit the needs of the child and his family. They are much more effective if used in conjunction with medication, since combined treatments are often superior to any single form of management. Behavioural and other psychological methods require a proper understanding about the nature of ADD, careful planning, monitoring and regular review of his behaviour and progress.

These methods must be adhered to and be carried out in a consistent manner. They may be time consuming but they often result in major gains for the child and his family when carried out properly.

CHAPTER 14

EDUCATIONAL STRATEGIES

> **Summary**
>
> Teachers need to appreciate the difficulties experienced by the child with ADD so that they make the necessary adjustments to the class environment.
>
> Teachers, parents and the child need to work as a team.
>
> Specific target behaviours need to be identified so that appropriate methods may be used to help the child improve his self-control in these areas.

Chapter 14 : Educational Strategies

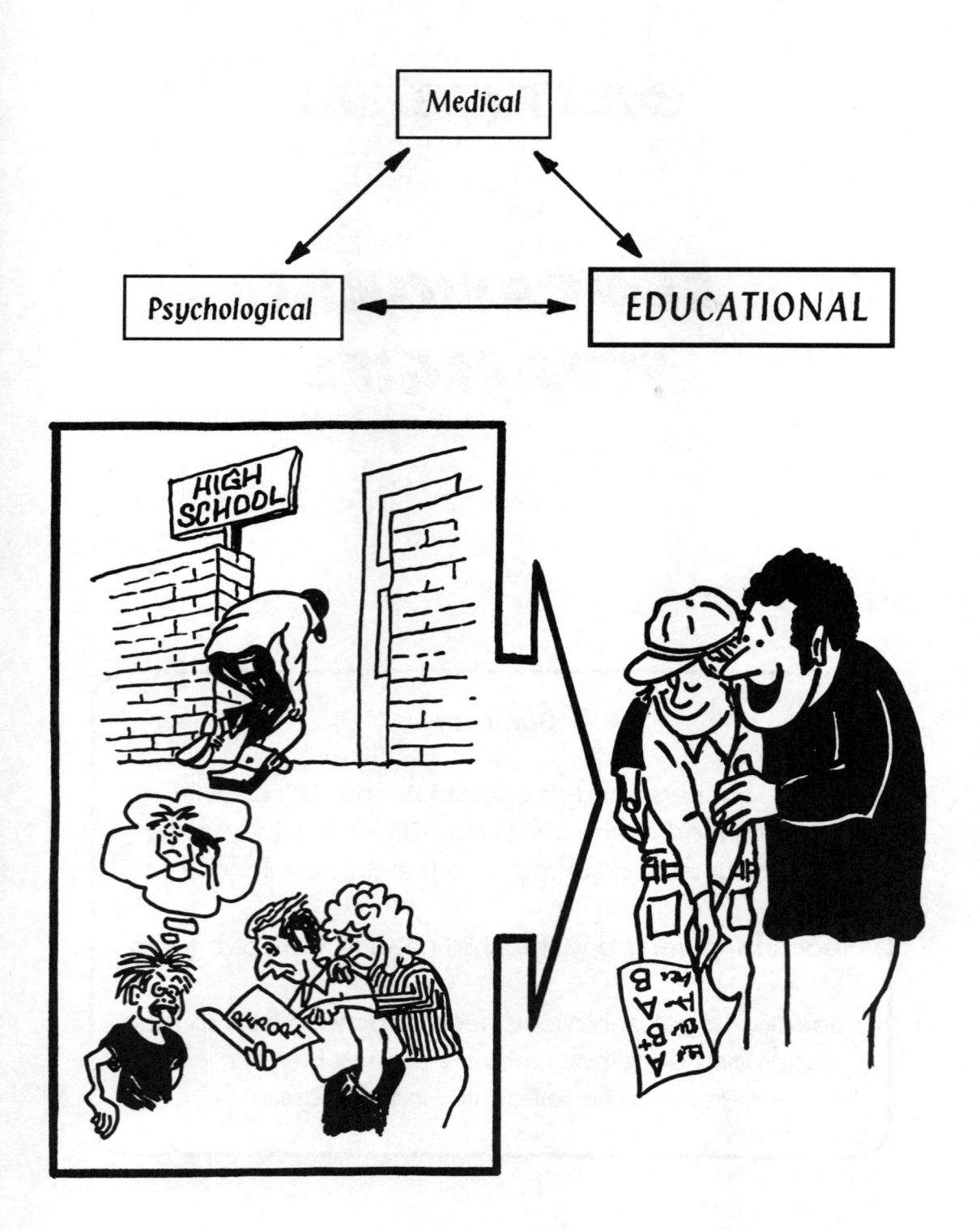

```
                    ┌──────────┐
                    │ Medical  │
                    └──────────┘
                    ↗          ↖
                   ↙            ↘
   ┌───────────────┐          ┌──────────────┐
   │ Psychological │ ←──────→ │ EDUCATIONAL  │
   └───────────────┘          └──────────────┘
```

116

Chapter 14 : Educational Strategies

Common Teacher Comments

The child with ADD comes to the attention of teachers as a result of the various difficulties he experiences in his learning, behaviour, social interactions and self esteem. It is very common to note certain remarks made by teachers, either verbally or in school reports: 'must learn to concentrate'; 'makes careless errors'; 'very easily distracted'; 'rarely completes his work'; 'disruptive in class'; 'untidy work habits'; 'disorganised'; 'unpopular with other students in the class'; 'inconsistent performance'; 'capable of doing much better work'; 'doesn't pay attention'; 'constantly in trouble in the school yard'; or 'needs to repeat this grade'. These comments are all very descriptive of children with ADD.

The child with ADD(+H) whose hyperactive and aggressive behaviour can be disruptive to the class soon comes to the notice of his teachers. Unfortunately, the quiet and well-behaved child with ADD(-H), who has difficulties in focusing and sustaining attention, may go unnoticed.

The Role Of Teachers

The child with ADD can be greatly supported when appropriate interventions are introduced by his teachers. Teachers need to view the child's functioning in all areas, including his academic performance, behaviour, self-esteem and social interactions. These areas must not be viewed in isolation since any one of them may directly influence the others. For example, his difficulties in learning may ultimately result in poor self-esteem or frustration which may aggravate the problems he has in controlling his behaviour and interacting with teachers and other students.

Interventions require careful planning and need to focus on both prevention of problem areas as well as the management of various behaviours when they occur. It is vital that his teachers understand the nature of ADD and become aware of the necessary and potentially helpful interventions.

Support for classroom teachers is vital, and it is highly desirable that the disorder is recognised by their colleagues and superiors. These include psychologists or guidance officers, student counsellors, special education teachers, speech pathologists as well as school medical and nursing staff. Such support staff can advise teachers in specific areas of management and may be invaluable in the professional development of teachers who necessarily have to work with students who have ADD in the classroom.

Teachers need to determine the behavioural and learning styles of the child with ADD, and those situations in which his various difficulties are likely to occur. This requires careful observation and monitoring of the child. Cooperation and collaboration with his parents is vital in devising practical programs for use at home and at school. A consistent approach by parents and teachers is vital.

Difficulties At School

The child with ADD very often experiences a range of difficulties at school. He is more likely to underachieve than other children. Schoolwork is often difficult for him because of his problems with selective and sustained attention, motivation and difficulties with persistence of effort and in staying on task.

He is also placed at a disadvantage because of his poor organisational skills, difficulties in starting and persisting with certain tasks and his variable and erratic performance. He produces less quality work than other students.

These problems are likely to result in messy and untidy schoolwork, poor ability to complete schoolwork and assignments, difficulties in following instructions, and a poor understanding and recall of relevant information. The outcomes of these difficulties include avoidance of schoolwork, underachievement and school refusal. He knows that he should do better, but he cannot understand why schoolwork is so difficult.

These academic difficulties may be further complicated if he has a coexisting specific learning disability, a situation which is more common in children with ADD than other students. The attentional problems caused by his ADD are likely to aggravate any associated learning difficulty.

The child with ADD(+H) often has additional complications because of his poor ability to control his behaviour, especially in social interactions in the classroom

Chapter 14 : Educational Strategies

and school yard. His inadvertent, but aggressive, disruptive and unacceptable behaviours are very likely to make him unpopular. His classmates are likely to retaliate, tease and reject him. Such responses from others may easily cause him to become isolated. His poor self-esteem is likely to deteriorate further.

Intervention Issues

His teacher needs to understand the subject of ADD and how the condition may affect him in various school-related activities. Any school-based program is likely to be more effective when employed in conjunction with medication and psychological strategies. Research shows that combined interventions are far superior to any single form of management. School programs are based on very similar principles described in the previous chapter.

It is vital that teachers work together with the child and his parents as a team. Contact with the other professionals involved in his management for example, his paediatrician, may be necessary from time to time. The child who has ADD benefits greatly from regularity, routine and consistency as part of an overall strategy. Clear and realistic expectations must be set and need to involve the child, parents and teachers.

Basic Concepts

In view of his difficulties with selective and sustained attention, problems with motivation, the need for immediate feedback, and his tendency to become rapidly accustomed or habituated to rewards and consequences, teachers need to devise programs and situations which take these issues into account.

It is important to monitor his behaviour and level of attention frequently. Positive feedback for acceptable behaviour, effort and performance must be given immediately. This principle also holds true when the various consequences for unacceptable behaviour are administered. Combinations of strategies need to be used at the same time. Some of these include the use of praise for positive behaviour, ignoring minor infringements, and dispensing reprimands for significant unacceptable behaviour.

Instructions must be brief, clearly stated and need to be given frequently. Class rules should be made obvious and preferably exhibited visually in a prominent place and in a colourful style. He needs to be regularly reminded of these rules and instructions.

Feedback and consequences are much more likely to be effective when they are given frequently and dispensed immediately. Teachers must deliver such feedback in a consistent way. Consequences need to be sufficiently powerful and relevant in order to influence his motivation to carry out necessary tasks, because he is often far less responsive to the usual incentives that work for other children.

The child with ADD quickly becomes accustomed to the same rewards if these are continued for too long. He is likely to lose interest in them, and they tend to become less effective over time. It is often useful to change incentives and rewards frequently to reduce the possibility of habituation to any single reward.

The more difficult, complex and tedious tasks which require sustained attention need to be organised and divided into smaller segments, and instructions need to be given clearly. Such tedious activities are best carried out in the morning when his difficulties with attention are likely to be less of a problem. He should be praised and reinforced during tasks and when they are completed. Physical exercise carried out during the day, particularly between more formal school tasks and in the afternoon, is often of great benefit.

Planning And Anticipation

It is often possible to reduce the likelihood of his inappropriate behaviour. His teachers need to plan ahead and pay particular attention to those situations which may trigger difficulties for him. He is likely to experience problems during transitions in activities. He needs to be made aware of any forthcoming activity several times before the transition takes place. He must be reminded of the rules of expected behaviour on a regular basis. He also needs to be reminded about the rewards and consequences which apply in each new situation.

Chapter 14 : Educational Strategies

Potential Problems With Other Students

His inappropriate behaviour can have major negative effects in various school settings. His difficulties with self-control may create disruption and may interfere with the activities of the other students. This is likely to provoke his classmates to laugh, tease or respond in other negative ways. These responses are likely to promote his unacceptable behaviour. Alternatively, they may retaliate or take revenge and so maintain his undesirable behaviour.

His classmates can assist their teacher by learning to ignore his unacceptable behaviour and by praising his more positive behaviour. This should reduce the likelihood of the repetition of his less desirable behaviour. Providing him with a suitable role model or 'buddy' who sits next to him, and who may provide him with appropriate feedback and praise, can also be a very useful strategy.

Treatment Targets

Before instituting practical programs or strategies to assist the child with ADD, teachers need to determine the specific difficulties he is experiencing. Among the common targets for intervention are: disruptiveness in the classroom; off-task behaviour; poor academic performance; unacceptable behaviour in the playground; difficulties with peer interactions; and poor self-esteem. Effective strategies should be aimed at the specific areas in which change is desired.

Teachers need to pay special attention to the problem areas and attempt to identify the triggers for his difficulties. They should also determine the methods they are currently using to manage him in the full range of tasks and situations. This should help teachers ascertain those types of rewards and consequences they are now using. They can determine the methods which are effective and those which may actually perpetuate his various difficulties.

It is important to identify alternative and more positive behaviours. He can learn these substitute behaviours so that they may replace the problem behaviours. His teachers must not assume that he automatically knows how to behave in different situations.

Chapter 14 : Educational Strategies

The various interventions which are about to be described are intended to increase the likelihood of success and help him reach his full potential. They cannot 'cure' his ADD. Even with the use of these methods it is possible that he may experience some difficulties from time to time. These interventions should also work very well with children who do not have ADD, since they are based on sound classroom practice.

Modifying The Classroom Environment

The child with ADD is at the whim of his immediate situation. He may have major difficulties in cooperating with and managing to follow through with instructions and tasks set by his teachers. Modifying the physical layout of the classroom in more appropriate ways will enable him to cope more effectively.

The traditional classroom is preferred to the open space classroom because it is less noisy and contains fewer visual and auditory distractions. It is more likely to improve his ability to stay on task and improve his self-control of behaviour.

Classroom activities need to be well organised, predictable and structured. It is desirable that he be informed about any forthcoming activities beforehand. A colourful visual display of class rules and a daily timetable in a prominent place is very helpful.

It is useful to sit him at a separate desk away from the other students in an area close to the teacher. This manoeuvre takes him away from his classmates who may otherwise reinforce his undesirable behaviour. It also enables the teacher to monitor his behaviour and also provide him with the necessary and frequent feedback and encouragement to stay on task. If he needs to sit next to another student, it is vital that the chosen student be a positive role model who may enhance the teacher's efforts.

Strategies To Improve His Attention

Introducing novel activities into the daily classroom activities is likely to improve his level of interest and the ability to selectively attend to his work. The different ways of doing this are listed in Appendix 7: 'Varying Learning Strategies'.

Chapter 14 : Educational Strategies

It is highly desirable that tasks and assignments be kept short. Any necessary lengthy projects should be broken down into bite-size pieces. He also needs to receive immediate feedback for each section of completed work.

Instructions are best given one at a time, and it is very important to check that he understands what is required of him. Teachers are able to assist by setting short-term goals and so improve his capacity to stay on task.

He is likely to experience greater success when teachers regularly monitor his effort and performance, and when they teach him appropriate self-monitoring skills. Instructions are more likely to be followed if they are given in combined verbal and written forms. Instructions need to be clear, unambiguous, concise and to the point.

It is useful to alternate the more intensive and monotonous tasks, which require sustained attention, with those that are likely to be of more interest to him such as physical activity. Computer programs generally promote his ability to focus and sustain attention extremely well, and this form of learning can be extremely useful for the child with ADD, far more so than the more formal lecture format. It is also useful if the teacher can match various academic activities and tasks with his abilities in each of the different areas of the curriculum.

Improving His Organisational And Planning Skills

Teachers may improve his ability with organisation by displaying and repeating basic work rules. He needs a notebook and diary in which he may enter details of important assignments, homework and messages for his parents. Teachers need to repeatedly check that the correct information is entered into these books. It is important that teachers and parents maintain close and frequent contact to discuss his assignments so that they can help him stay on track.

Regular supervision of his work enables teachers to check his understanding of the task or exercise at hand and its accuracy. He needs to be praised each time he carries out acceptable work. Teachers can help him focus on short-term goals so that he can carry out work in stages.

Chapter 14 : Educational Strategies

Helping Him Control His Behaviour

Teachers should try to ignore his minor infringements of behaviour and actively praise him immediately for positive behaviour. They should supervise him more closely during transitions or changes in class routine. If a significant behaviour problem occurs, teachers should be prepared and ensure that he receives an agreed-upon consequence, for example, the time out procedure. The use of reasoning, lecturing and criticism should be avoided at these times.

He needs to be taught some basic skills in self-monitoring of behaviour and to replace negative behaviours such as yelling with more appropriate methods such as putting up his hand. He should be praised each time these positive behaviours are carried out. A specific behavioural contract, which needs to be arranged between teachers, parents and himself, can be a very useful tool in helping him gain self-control over his behaviour.

Improving His Ability To Control Muscle Activity

The child with ADD(+H) can be very restless and this may be a distraction and irritation to teachers and other students. Teachers may assist by allowing him to stand at his desk when carrying out various tasks and encouraging short breaks between activities so that he may walk around or outside the classroom.

His activity level is likely to be more of a problem during transitions in activities. Teachers should supervise him more closely at those times when there is a change of venue and also during changes in schedule.

Helping Improve His Self-Esteem

The child with ADD is very prone to suffer from a poor self-esteem which is often aggravated by negative reactions and comments from other students. It is important to remember that many things are more difficult for the child with ADD. His positive behaviours must not be taken for granted. Teachers can help by providing regular and frequent encouragement and support. He needs to be praised for effort, suitable performance and work output. He should receive feedback for acceptable behaviour.

Chapter 14 : Educational Strategies

Teachers need to actively look for areas in which he is working well and praise his efforts, rather than focus solely on unacceptable aspects of his behaviour. Teachers and parents should regularly discuss his positive characteristics and determine ways in which the more difficult areas may be improved.

Teachers may arrange to spend special times to talk alone with him to discuss specific issues regarding academic work, behaviour and social interactions. Regular positive feedback is vital and he should be reinforced for all positive aspects of his school experience. Teachers may need to reduce his work load when his ability to stay on task wanes or when he is becoming stressed.

Improving His Interactions With Other Students

Teachers often find it very useful to monitor the ways he interacts with the other students. This requires careful observation of both positive and less successful relationships with different students. He should be rewarded for appropriate interactions. He may need to learn some basic social skills, and his teachers may do this in the context of a social training program in the classroom. He and his teachers may determine some specific social goals for him.

Allowing him to sit near favourable role models can be a very useful strategy. Teachers may arrange cooperative learning activities so that he has greater opportunities to work and interact with other students. This also enables him to learn useful social behaviours. He may also be given special responsibilities so that the other students may observe him carrying out such positive activities.

Additional Methods

His parents can help in a number of ways. Regular contact with his teachers will allow them to understand the type of work required of him and the homework he needs to carry out. A consistent approach between his parents and teachers is likely to improve and reinforce his progress in learning. The child and his parents may improve the learning environment at home by providing him with suitable study space, arranging set routines for study and helping him organise his diary, school bag, work books and other necessary equipment.

Chapter 14 : Educational Strategies

Computerised interactive educational programs and word processing can be highly useful because they improve his ability to focus and sustain attention. A low student-teacher ratio is best for the child with ADD.

The child who is underachieving may require special school-based programs or private tuition to enable him to catch up in any areas of weakness.

The issue of management of the various specific learning disabilities is beyond the scope of this book.

Traps To Avoid

The school management of the child with ADD can be stressful for his teachers. They need to understand his condition and use appropriate methods to assist in managing specific aspects of his ADD. Some teachers may not appreciate how he differs from other children. They may inadvertently use methods which are unlikely to help. In fact, they may actually aggravate his difficulties and add to their own frustrations.

Traps which teachers need to avoid are: using negative labels and put-downs; increasing their interactions with him when they should ignore his minor infringements of behaviour; using force and a domineering stance; ignoring his more positive behaviours and interactions with others; ignoring his learning and academic progress and concentrating only on his unacceptable behaviours and interactions with other students; refusing to accept that he has a true disability which requires some specific interventions; and not working closely with his parents.

CHAPTER 15

THE FUTURE OF CHILDREN WITH ATTENTION DEFICIT DISORDER

Summary

Many children with ADD outgrow their disability by their late teenage years.

Some children develop complications and these include academic underachievement, poor social interactions, personal stress, oppositional defiant disorder and conduct disorder. These may be prevented with proper assessment and early treatment.

A significant proportion of children continue their ADD symptoms into adult life.

Chapter 15: The Future Of Children With Attention Deficit Disorder

Many, But Not All, Children Outgrow Their ADD

It was once thought that all children with ADD outgrew their condition, but this is not the case. Although many children will outgrow their symptoms by their late teens, others are not so fortunate. Some children with ADD(+H) continue all their symptoms into adult life. Others continue to have difficulties in paying attention, but their problems in controlling muscle activity improve with age. Although estimates vary, between 30-50 per cent of children with ADD continue to show evidence of ADD as adults. It is difficult to accurately predict who will outgrow their disability.

A great deal of psychological harm may occur if his ADD is left untreated during childhood. It is wrong to assume that all his difficulties will be reversed by the time he reaches his teenage years and that he will automatically grow out of it unscathed. Even if his ADD improves over time, it is highly possible that he will be left with deep psychological scars that will need healing later in life.

Many children with ADD have a very unfortunate history of failure and develop a poor self-esteem and many other drawbacks from their very early lives, and into primary school and then secondary school. If practical methods are not introduced during these vulnerable years, a number of serious complications may result. These are usually preventable with appropriate management.

Factors Which Affect The Outcome Of Children With ADD

The outcome of children with ADD depends on several important factors. The outlook for any child is likely to be worse if many of these risk factors impinge on him. Conversely, if there are fewer risk factors acting on the child, the outcome is likely to be more positive.

Some of the adverse factors which may affect the future of the child with ADD are: the more severe type of the condition; diagnosis and commencement of treatment at a relatively late age; the presence of associated conditions, for example, specific learning disabilities; the presence of complications such as underachievement at school; an imperfect understanding of ADD by parents or teachers; the child's refusal to accept that he has a real disability; severe family stress, poor family functioning or a lack of support from other family members; major marital difficulties; the presence of other children with ADD or any other disability; poor relationship between parents and the child with ADD; physical or emotional problems, such as ADD or a depressive illness, affecting one or both parents; and negative relationships between teachers, classmates and the child with ADD.

These factors need to be considered before treatment is commenced. Some of these may be reversed with appropriate management in their own right, and once these factors are corrected there is a greater probability that the overall outcome will be improved.

Academic Underachievement

The child with ADD is very likely to underachieve at school as a direct result of his difficulties with selective and sustained attention. This often results in gaps in his knowledge in many critical areas of academic work. His understanding of the basic academic skills may be lacking, in spite of normal intelligence.

His underachievement shows itself in unsatisfactory comments and results in school reports. He may be asked to repeat one or more grades throughout his school career, the notion being that he needs to 'catch up'. His problems at school may be aggravated if he has a coexistent specific learning disability such as a reading, writing or arithmetic disorder.

If he experiences very great academic difficulties, the child with ADD may fail to develop adequate literacy or numeracy skills and may ultimately fail at school, dropping out of the educational system altogether.

The Stress Of Having ADD

The child with ADD often experiences major problems with self-confidence and poor self-esteem. If he has suffered repeated failure in a variety of areas, for example at school and in his social interactions, it is possible that he may even develop a depressive illness.

ADD can create considerable stress and he may experience a range of stress-related symptoms such as anxiety and a general inability to cope with various aspects of his life. As they grow older, some children with ADD may become involved in substance abuse including excessive intake of alcohol, nicotine or even illicit drugs, in an attempt to cope with their stress.

Family Stress

Family stress is a very common occurrence in the family of a child with ADD. This may show itself in a number of ways including: injury to the child with ADD, either accidental or non-accidental; negative interactions with his brothers and sisters; and chronic anxiety, depression, psychosomatic and other symptoms of stress affecting the parents. Such stress may contribute to marital problems, breakdown and divorce.

Some parents may experience considerable hardship in their attempt to cope with a child who finds it difficult to control his behaviour. They may think that they have run out of all options available to them and feel that they have exhausted their energy and resources. If the parents can cope no further, some may force the child to leave home and he may become a street kid. This is quite likely to contribute to a poor outcome and future.

Social Difficulties

The child with ADD(+H) has poor self-control of behaviour which can lead to various difficulties in interacting with other people. If he experiences repeated conflicts with his peers, he is very likely to have difficulties in making friends and in maintaining friendships. His behaviour is likely to get him into constant trouble in the classroom or school yard and such infringements may result in repeated detentions, suspensions or even expulsion from school if he constantly breaks class rules and school regulations.

He may also have problems in relating to children outside school and this often makes it difficult for him to form positive, worthwhile and rewarding relationships. Such difficulties are likely to worsen his poor self-esteem. As he grows older, his poor social skills are likely to result in a poor social adjustment in the wider world.

Chapter 15: The Future Of Children With Attention Deficit Disorder

Oppositional Defiant Disorder

His poor self-control often results in increasing difficulties in the way he interacts with his parents and teachers. They may attempt to control his behaviour by using increasing negative and more forceful or aggressive methods. Over time these interactions may result in Oppositional Defiant Disorder (ODD).

In ODD he demonstrates oppositional, negative, spiteful and defiant behaviour. Although his behaviour shows itself in verbal hostility, he is not usually physically aggressive.

He is often argumentative and oppositional at home and sometimes at school. His behaviour may later become a problem in other settings as well. He does not usually admit to being difficult, and instead blames others for causing him to do the things he is being accused of. He often justifies what he has done and does not accept his part in it.

ODD typically starts before puberty. His self-esteem is usually quite poor and he is rather moody. He is very easily frustrated and temper tantrums are common. Some children with ODD go on to develop Conduct Disorder.

The common symptoms of ODD include: frequent loss of temper; often argues with adults; repeatedly blames others; easily annoyed by others; frequently angry and hostile; deliberately annoys others; often spiteful; repeatedly swears and puts other people down; and often refuses to carry out adult requests, for example, house work and other chores.

Conduct Disorder

The main focus of this condition is a repeated tendency to infringe the basic rights of other people. He refuses to accept or obey the rules of society. This pattern of behaviour is carried out at home, at school and in the community.

Conduct Disorder often starts before puberty. He lacks a conscience and does not seem to show any concerns for the feelings of others. He feels little, if any, guilt, remorse or regret after he carries out his aggressive acts.

Chapter 15: The Future Of Children With Attention Deficit Disorder

In spite of his bravado and 'tough guy' image, his self esteem is usually poor. He is also quite irritable and easily frustrated when he does not get his own way, throwing temper outbursts with little provocation. He is usually anxious and has a tendency to become depressed. His school progress is often poor and his skills with reading and writing are below those of other young people.

Because of his antisocial behaviour and repeated violation of rules, he may be suspended from school or be 'kicked out of home' and become a 'street kid'. He may get into trouble with the police. His parents may arrange foster care for him because they can no longer cope. Alternatively, he may be committed to an institution if the problem is extreme.

There is a possibility that he will become involved in the illicit drug culture. This use of drugs may result in addiction. He may be involved in fights and this can result in physical injuries. He may be sexually promiscuous and may contract a sexually transmitted disease. An unwanted pregnancy may also be the result of his impulsive sexual behaviour.

The outcome varies. His behaviour may improve with time and as he matures. However, he may continue his unlawful activities into adult life and develop a true antisocial personality and continue his behaviour, possibly getting into later trouble with the police and the legal system.

The common signs of conduct disorder include: repeated stealing and lying; running away from home; deliberate fire setting; truanting from school; breaking and entering; destroying property; cruelty to animals; using weapons in fights; forcing others to have sex with him; starting fights with others; physical cruelty to people; and mugging or armed robbery.

Adult Attention Deficit Disorder

As mentioned previously, not all children outgrow their disability. A significant number of children with ADD continue to experience various difficulties in their adult lives. The symptoms of adult ADD are similar to those observed in children, although it varies considerably in severity from one person to another.

Chapter 15: The Future Of Children With Attention Deficit Disorder

Common behaviours and symptoms experienced by adults with ADD include: difficulty in focusing or sustaining attention on tasks; poor persistence with tasks requiring effort; forgetfulness; being easily distracted; restlessness; impulsiveness; temper outbursts; unpredictable behaviour; anxiety; depression; and sleep disturbance. Not all of these symptoms need to be present to make a diagnosis.

Many adults with this condition are currently misdiagnosed and may be treated for other conditions such as depression, panic attacks and other psychiatric disorders. It is hoped that the diagnosis of adult ADD will become increasingly recognised so that more appropriate and effective methods of management are introduced to assist the sufferers of this disorder.

Adults with ADD may also have difficulties in their interactions with other adults including various family members, friends and in more intimate relationships. Their condition often imposes considerable stress on these other people.

Some adults with ADD are more than likely to have difficulties with employment. Their underachievement at school may adversely affect gaining appropriate qualifications for subsequent employment and career pursuits. Difficulties in sustaining attention may make it difficult for them to succeed in certain occupations. Problems in self-control may create difficulties in their interactions with their work mates and colleagues. Some adults with ADD move from one job to another as a result of their difficulties with self-control and impulsiveness.

Chapter 16 : Facts And Fallacies About Attention Deficit Disorder

CHAPTER 16

FACTS AND FALLACIES ABOUT ATTENTION DEFICIT DISORDER

> **Summary**
>
> Some of the available information about ADD is inaccurate.
>
> Several of these common myths and misconceptions are summarised and addressed.

Chapter 16 : Facts And Fallacies About Attention Deficit Disorder

Facts And Fallacies

There are many misconceptions and fallacies about ADD. These may lead parents to seek assessments and treatments which are quite inappropriate and unsuitable. They may also bring about a range of negative emotions and false hopes, and create poor communication and a lack of cooperation between the child with ADD, his parents, brothers, sisters and teachers.

Some of the common myths about ADD will be stated and each will be followed by more correct and accurate information. Many of these points have already been covered throughout this book. It is worthwhile repeating them because such fallacies are still frequently communicated and need to be dispelled.

Myth

ADD is caused by poor parenting.

Fact

ADD is a biological problem that affects a particular part of the brain. It shows up as difficulties in controlling his behaviour and problems in paying attention. The symptoms are variable and unpredictable. The usual methods of discipline which work for other children are far less likely to be effective when applied to the child with ADD. Some people may not realise that his disability makes him different to other children. To make matters worse, other people may blame the parents for their 'poor parenting' because they cannot control him.

The child with ADD, and particularly ADD(+H), can be very difficult to manage in many areas, and most parents would be exasperated by the day to day, week to week, month to month difficulties imposed on them by his poor self-control of behaviour. Their parenting skills, which are suitable for other children, may not be effective when applied to the child with ADD. Poor parenting is not the cause of ADD. Rather, the pressures imposed on his parents often makes their job of parenting very difficult.

Chapter 16 : Facts And Fallacies About Attention Deficit Disorder

Myth

Children with ADD can always control their behaviour and pay attention.

Fact

His difficulties with self-control and self-motivation are likely to result in variable effort and erratic performance, as well as difficulties in managing various tasks and activities. His disability also affects the way he interacts with other people. The physiological problem which affects a part of his brain is greatly influenced by the various situations in which he finds himself. On occasions he can perform certain tasks very well, whereas at other times he may carry out the same activities very poorly. This is often mistaken as 'laziness' or 'naughtiness'.

But he is not naughty or lazy. He simply lacks the self-control needed to carry out various activities in a consistent way. There are many things he can do well, provided the setting is one which provides him with the necessary conditions which enable him to overcome the difficulties he experiences in self-control of behaviour and attention. Appropriate treatment 'normalises' the function of his brain's self-control mechanism, and provides him with the opportunity to carry out various tasks in a more controlled fashion.

◊◊◊◊◊◊◊◊◊

Myth

All children with ADD are hyperactive.

Fact

Not all children with ADD are hyperactive. Some professionals, unfortunately, rely on the presence of overactivity to make the diagnosis of ADD. As a result, some children with ADD are not identified, and this may lead to an inappropriate diagnosis and ineffective treatments.

Chapter 16 : Facts And Fallacies About Attention Deficit Disorder

Children with ADD(-H), or ADD without hyperactivity, show little, if any evidence of hyperactivity or impulsiveness. Many of them respond to medication which often results in significant improvements in their ability to pay attention, school progress and self-esteem.

The message, then, is quite clear. Hyperactivity is not a necessary criterion for diagnosing ADD. On the other hand, any child who is experiencing any difficulty in focusing or sustaining attention must be considered as suffering from possible ADD.

◊◊◊◊◊◊◊◊◊

Myth

ADD only affects children.

Fact

Contrary to previous thinking, not all children outgrow their disability. In fact, as many as 50 per cent of children continue to have various difficulties into adult life. This may affect many aspects of their lives. Many of them are also left with the legacy of learning difficulties, poor self-esteem and other psychological disorders and difficulties in maintaining positive relationships.

The medical treatment of adult ADD is similar to that of ADD in children. A major problem for adult sufferers is that their condition is often not recognised for what it really is. As a result they may be treated for other emotional problems such as depression or anxiety disorders.

It is hoped that this situation will change as the diagnosis of adult ADD becomes increasingly accepted and recognised as a clinical entity by professionals who are involved in the management of psychological difficulties in adults. Adults with ADD will then be managed with the use of appropriate interventions.

◊◊◊◊◊◊◊◊◊

Chapter 16 : Facts And Fallacies About Attention Deficit Disorder

Myth

ADD is uncommon in girls.

Fact

It is true that ADD is more frequently diagnosed in boys, partly because they display hyperactivity, impulsiveness and various 'behaviour problems' more readily than girls. However, the number of girls affected is significant, but many of them are not identified because they may do not demonstrate the difficult or disruptive behaviours that are displayed by boys with ADD(+H).

It is a fact that the hyperactivity of boys with ADD(+H) tends to improve with age. Interestingly, the number of men and women with adult ADD is about the same. This indicates that, as their hyperactivity improves, many men with ADD are left with a similar picture to women with ADD.

◊◊◊◊◊◊◊◊◊

Myth

ADD is like any other type of learning disability and should be treated as such.

Fact

ADD is not the same as a specific learning disability. A true learning disability is the result of a developmental problem in processing information and deriving meaning from such information. ADD, on the other hand, results in poor control of attention and behaviour. Certainly, most children who have 'pure' ADD are at a considerable disadvantage and they often underachieve at school, but this is the direct result of their problems with attention.

To add to this confusion, the child with ADD is more likely to have an associated specific learning disability than other children. It is important that he receives a proper assessment of his ADD, which is best treated with medication.

Chapter 16 : Facts And Fallacies About Attention Deficit Disorder

Once his poor attention is improved with medication, more deliberate observations of his academic skills and progress can be instituted. If this manoeuvre does not bring about a great improvement, a formal educational assessment needs to be performed, to check for the potential presence of a specific learning disability. It is vital to consider the possible coexistence of ADD, of course, which needs treatment in its own right. If this is the case, his learning disability must not be managed in isolation because only a partial improvement will take place.

◊◊◊◊◊◊◊◊◊

Myth

The label of Attention Deficit Disorder is harmful to children with the disorder.

Fact

In general, negative labels can be very harmful when applied to any child, and this can be a particular problem for the child with ADD. On the other hand, the 'label', or rather the correct diagnosis, of ADD is often a very positive statement in that it helps explain the reasons for the many difficulties he experiences.

Many parents are relieved when they discover that ADD is a disability which is treatable. The diagnosis is not a harmful 'label' if the condition is fully explained to the child and his parents, and is understood and accepted by them.

◊◊◊◊◊◊◊◊◊

Myth

Medication is the only form of treatment available to children with ADD.

Fact

Medications are a very important form of treatment. They have been proven to be highly effective in most children with ADD. The child who suffers from mild ADD may benefit from medication as the only form of treatment.

Chapter 16 : Facts And Fallacies About Attention Deficit Disorder

Medication normalises the activity and function of the poorly operating area of the brain. This 'correction' enables him to improve self-control and enhances his ability to focus and sustain attention.

On the other hand, another child may experience various other difficulties and these need to be assessed and treated in their own right. For example he may have a combination of a specific learning difficulty, difficulties with muscle co-ordination, bedwetting and oppositional behaviour.

The assessment of these are best considered after his ADD has been properly controlled with medication. Specific psychological and educational strategies may be necessary in order to assist the child who suffers from these coexisting disabilities, but these are best carried out in conjunction with medication.

◊◊◊◊◊◊◊◊◊

Myth

ADD is caused by food allergies.

Fact

There is no scientific proof which shows that allergies or sensitivities to various foods, colourings, preservatives, additives or natural salicylates are the causes of ADD. A very small proportion of parents of children with ADD swear that their child has a sensitivity to sugar and are convinced that a reduction in his sugar intake has a beneficial effect. If this is the case, parents need to be supported in their efforts. They need to be provided with up-to-date information about the proven methods of treatment so that they are in a better position to make an informed decision about management.

In general, however, dietary interventions are not useful in most cases of ADD and are not usually recommended.

◊◊◊◊◊◊◊◊◊

Chapter 17: Future Directions

CHAPTER 17

FUTURE DIRECTIONS

> **Summary**
>
> Several different avenues are likely to improve the lives of children with ADD and their families and to prevent potential complications.
>
> They include: research; community and professional education; early identification and treatment; support groups and advocacy.

Chapter 17 : Future Directions

Research

As a result of ongoing research, we have gained a much clearer understanding of ADD, its causes and various treatments. This research has been carried out in laboratories and in the community. Its practical application to children and families has enabled us to accept the condition for what it really is. People are now realising that children with ADD suffer from a true disability; they are not 'problem children', but rather 'children with a problem'.

Further research into the various aspects of ADD will eventually pay dividends. Avenues for further investigation include: the genetics of ADD; the chemistry and physiology of specific areas and connections in the brain; the development of more accurate and sensitive assessment and diagnostic criteria; and development, application and modification of different treatment strategies involving medication, educational and psychological methods.

We will ultimately be in a more favourable position to offer a range of improved preventive strategies and more accurate assessment and effective treatment. Genetic counselling and early intervention may become increasingly possible, and these may improve the outlook of children with the condition.

The differences between ADD(+H) and ADD(-H) should become more clear in the near future and the diagnosis of the more subtle form, ADD(-H), will be more readily made. This should result in earlier identification and improved management of the condition, as well as preventing academic underachievement and emotional difficulties in children who suffer from ADD(-H).

ADD in adults is a new and very challenging area for research. With improved diagnostic criteria and experience with various treatment methods, the quality in the lives of these adults may be significantly improved.

Practical research into the causes of the various associated problems will lead to improved methods of intervention in the areas of specific learning disabilities and Tourette Syndrome. The relationship between depressive illness and ADD is another field of research. The management of the important complications, oppositional defiant and conduct disorders can be very difficult, and clinical research into these entities may provide us with more effective treatments.

Chapter 17: Future Directions

Community Awareness And Professional Development

Some parents of children with ADD do not understand the condition and they are poorly informed about the necessary methods and special skills which are needed to manage their child's condition. This same problem also exists in the general community in which there is often a poor availability of accurate and up-to-date information about the condition.

The topic of ADD appears regularly in the media. In general, this is a valuable exercise because it increases community awareness. Unfortunately, some of the information presented on the radio, television, magazines, and newspapers focuses on the extreme forms of deviant behaviour, for example aggression, of children with severe ADD(+H). It may ignore the less obvious problems of underachievement and poor self-esteem of those children with ADD(-H).

Accurate information must be presented to the child and parents so that they may make informed decisions about the various treatment options. The media is a powerful instrument for disseminating information, but it must be provided with appropriate information in order to get the right messages across.

Other ways of communicating information is through books and other written materials available through various outlets including libraries, book shops and ADD Support Groups. Experts on the subject of ADD may be invited to speak to a variety of audiences and inform them about the condition.

Because ADD is a common condition, it would be appropriate that trainees and undergraduate students receive relevant training in this area if there is a likelihood that they will be working with families and children with ADD in the future. This strategy could prevent and reduce considerable suffering in such families.

In a similar way, professionals who are already working in the health, education and welfare areas may not have received training in ADD. They may need to learn specific skills in assessing and managing children with this condition, and this requires professional development with the backing and support of their supervisors. This will enable these workers to be an integral part of a treatment team and assist parents in devising relevant programs to help their children.

Chapter 17 : Future Directions

Early Identification And Intervention

ADD is a chronic disability which may result in a range of complications if it is not managed properly. The future and outcome for many children with untreated ADD may be quite poor. It is far better to identify children with ADD early in their lives so that the necessary and effective treatments may be instituted, enabling them to take increasing control of their situation. This is likely to prevent many of the potential negative outcomes for children and their families.

Early identification and intervention naturally requires that relevant professionals who work with children and families become versed in the many aspects of the condition. Community health and educational organisations need to consider the various ways in which they can train their workers in the area of ADD. They also need to consider ways in which to provide the necessary services to meet the needs of these children and families.

ADD Support Groups

Some parents of children with ADD develop informal networks with other parents who find themselves in a similar situation. Such efforts enable them to support one another and offer valuable advice. These local liaisons can bring about many positive changes. They include: a better understanding of these children; the sharing of useful and practical ideas and methods; the distribution of current and practical information and other resources; and the promotion of useful and empathic friendships.

Many parents who have children with ADD feel isolated and vulnerable, and other parents who can empathise with and understand their predicament are able to offer the support which most professionals cannot provide. Parents can empower each other by sharing useful practical information, communicating and providing support at all times, but particularly during times of crisis.

As a result of these processes, some parents are now developing more formal associations or ADD Support Groups. These groups are usually set up in order to address the various problems, and find practical solutions for their own personal situation. The ways in which this is being carried out include a very broad range of skills and strategies such as: communicating and participating; planning, decision making, and leadership; and establishing acceptance and trust within the group.

When they operate in positive and effective ways, these groups may provide a range of services including: extending support for other parents of children with ADD; increasing community awareness by becoming involved with the media; arranging forums and discussions with experts in the field; empowering people with information; and distributing relevant literature about ADD and its related conditions. They may also refer families to appropriate assessment and treatment services. The specific functions of each ADD Support Group need to be determined by its members.

Advocacy

The issue of advocacy for children with ADD, their families and teachers is a very sensitive but important area which is being addressed more openly and more frequently. Advocacy may take place at several different levels, from the school face and local community level to the much broader organisational, administrative and political spheres.

Support groups and various professional bodies may lobby various decision makers for a range of human resources, facilities and funding with the aim of providing appropriate diagnostic and management services for children and others involved in their care. The various professionals who are involved in the management of children with ADD need to ask: 'what strategies are needed for relevant people to act as true advocates for these children, their families and their teachers so that they, the children, can become more effective people who reach their potential ?'

APPENDICES

1	Specific Behavioural Aspects Of ADD	151
2	Assessment - Issues For Parents	157
3	Assessment - Teacher Issues	163
4	Benefits Of Medication	167
5	Some Specific Psychological Strategies	169
6	Skills Development	179
7	Varying Learning Strategies	183

APPENDIX 1

SPECIFIC BEHAVIOURAL ASPECTS OF ADD

Appendix 1 presents some of the interpretations people use to describe the various symptoms and behaviours of children with ADD. Some of the consequences of these behaviours are also outlined.

Poor selective attention and sustained attention are often interpreted as:

- Easily distracted
- Switching off
- Attention drifts off
- Loses meaning of conversations
- Difficulty in following discussions
- Focuses on unimportant things
- Forgets important messages
- Eyes roam aimlessly
- Poor concentration
- Difficulty in paying attention
- Daydreaming
- Doesn't listen properly
- Instructions need to be repeated
- Difficulty in focusing
- Forgets what needs to be done
- Loose thought patterns
- Skips words or sentences

Consequences for the child:

- Emotional - feeling embarrassed, humiliated, helpless and isolated
- Spoken information doesn't make sense to him
- He finds it difficult to work out what is going on
- He has difficulty in following verbal instructions
- His responses may have nothing to do with the topic under discussion
- Poor comprehension and understanding of tasks and instructions
- He does not develop a full idea of what is being said and is likely to miss out on important items of information

Appendix 1 : Specific Behavioural Aspects Of ADD

Consequences of his poor attention for others:

- Parents and teachers becomes increasingly frustrated with him
- Teachers reprimand him for carelessness and errors
- He may be labelled as 'careless', 'stupid', 'lazy' or 'irresponsible'

Problems in planning, editing or monitoring behaviour are often interpreted as:

- Does not use information in a worthwhile manner
- Responds to questions in unpredictable and often incorrect ways
- Loses his train of thought when responding to questions
- Often misplaces or loses things
- Work is often careless with mistakes eg in spelling, writing and calculations
- Takes inappropriate short cuts when carrying out work activities and tasks
- Applies the least amount of effort and time, especially when it comes to 'boring' tasks or those that require sustained attention
- Difficulty in keeping track of assignments or projects
- Has difficulties in keeping his room, desk or clothing tidy and orderly
- Difficulty in keeping things together in groups eg books on shelves
- Does not keep his schoolwork organised in notebooks, folders or files
- His sense of time is unrealistic
- Problems in managing his own money
- His learning is often based on trial and error

Consequences:

- Makes repeated promises to do better but these often fail
- Needs to be supervised closely and reminded to carry out tasks
- His performance is better in one-to-one situations
- Difficulty in participating in class discussions
- May lose interest in certain tasks or activities
- Schoolwork may seem pointless to him
- He becomes easily bored with work that requires sustained attention
- Poor academic progress and underachievement
- Self-esteem may deteriorate as a result of repeated failure

Appendix 1 : Specific Behavioural Aspects Of ADD

- His life may lack continuity because he cannot connect what is happening in the present with what has happened previously or what is likely to follow
- Difficulty in learning rules, planning ahead and organising himself
- Difficulty in starting certain tasks and in persisting with the task at hand
- Does not complete tasks and is likely to jump from one thing to another
- Difficulties in knowing how to respond appropriately to new situations and how to change behaviour accordingly
- Continually surprised by each task requirement, no matter how many times he has performed it previously
- Often runs late for class and other activities
- Forgets what he needs to take to class or what he needs to do homework
- Often forgets what needs to be done at school or for homework
- Often leaves things behind at home or at school
- May lose his assignment sheets or diary

Problems in inhibiting motor activity is often interpreted as:

- Overactive or 'always on the go'
- Goes from one thing to another
- Can't sit still
- Clumsy
- Runs rather than walks
- Needs to touch or handle things
- Talks excessively to too loudly
- Restless or fidgety
- Acts as if driven by a motor
- Climbs excessively
- Restless during sleep
- Can't leave people alone
- Out of his seat a lot of the time
- Squirmy

Consequences:

These behaviours are likely to irritate other people because they are often very annoying, distracting and disruptive. His school mates and other children may retaliate in negative and aggressive ways, and he may be subjected to ridicule and scapegoating. This aspect of behaviour may also result in physical injury such as lacerations, bruising and more serious injuries such as head trauma, particularly if he is also very impulsive.

Appendix 1 : Specific Behavioural Aspects Of ADD

Poor self-control or poor regulation of behaviour

The child with ADD(+H) often has great difficulty in taking control of his general behaviour, finding it difficult to inhibit important aspects of behaviour when the situation requires him to do so. This is especially a problem during transitions, when it is necessary for him to go from one activity to another. Such poor control can result in the following :

- Does not plan ahead
- Hums or makes silly noises
- Does not think of consequences
- Cannot put off desires or wishes
- Fails to follow instructions
- Unpremeditated actions
- Does things without thinking
- Opts for immediate satisfaction
- Talks before thinking
- Impatient
- Intolerant
- Overly keen and eager
- Overly spontaneous
- Unpredictable behaviour
- Talking out of turn
- Acts on the spur of the moment
- Shows no 'common sense'
- Impulsive
- Reacts too quickly to situations
- Cannot stop impulses
- Does whatever comes to mind
- Gets things over and done with
- Urge to pull things apart
- Demanding
- Quick tempered
- 'Hot and cold'
- Rash and unconsidered actions

Consequences:

- Makes many silly and careless errors
- Can't set long-term goals nor work toward them
- Takes chances on a dare or a whim
- Careless damage of property, either his own or that of others
- Does not change behaviours that bother or offend other people
- Does not learn from experience
- Disorganised
- Failure to consider potentially serious or dangerous consequences
- Engages in frequent and unnecessary risk taking

Appendix 1 : Specific Behavioural Aspects Of ADD

Poor control of emotions (emotional disinhibition) results in:

- Emotions are always near the surface eg laughs too loudly, giggles too often, cries very easily or loses temper easily (short-tempered)
- Easily frustrated
- Easily triggered into aggressive or other negative emotional states
- Rapid mood swings and changes in emotions
- Demands immediate responses and rewards from other people
- Can become aggressive over minor incidents
- Complains or protests too frequently about unimportant matters
- Cannot tolerate being teased by others

Poor control of behaviour in social situations results in:

- Difficulty in waiting his turn in games
- Cannot share or cooperate with other children
- Does not pick up social cues, and may persist with inappropriate behaviour in spite of negative feedback
- Unkind to others, for example, berating or physically abusing them
- Interrupts the conversation of others
- Disruptive in a group situations
- Triggers conflict within a group
- Often makes indiscreet and inappropriate statements to others
- Keeps things 'stirred up' and does not know when to stop
- Unaware that he is being disruptive
- Acts in an egocentric way
- May make friends but loses them quickly

Consequences:

- Seeks the company of older or younger children
- Others view him as being immature, selfish and uncooperative
- Other children complain about his behaviour to the teacher
- Difficulty in being accepted as part of the group
- Others retaliate either verbally or physically

Appendix 1 : Specific Behavioural Aspects Of ADD

- Cannot compete successfully in team games
- Rejected, isolated and ostracised, eventually becoming a loner
- Poor self-esteem
- Acquires a bad reputation and receives negative labels from others
- Does not understand why he is so unpopular
- Retreats from peer interactions and may take up other interests

APPENDIX 2

ASSESSMENT - ISSUES FOR PARENTS

The following issues are important to consider in the assessment of the child with possible ADD. These matters may be raised during a direct interview with the parents, or they may be answered by means of a questionnaire which can be sent to the parents before the initial consultation.

Main concerns

What are the main concerns you have about your child ? Consider the following areas and describe your concerns in detail:

- behaviour
- general development
- physical health
- learning and academic progress
- self-esteem and emotional health
- relationships with other children
- relationships with mother, father, brothers and sisters

What are your ideas about the possible causes of his difficulties ?

Write down the possible reasons for his problems.

What are your concerns about his future ?

Write your comments about any concerns you have about his future ?

What are his positive qualities ?

Comment on his strengths, assets and any other positive characteristics which he shows from time to time.

Tests and investigations carried out previously

What tests, if any, have been carried out, approximately when, and what were the results ? (These may include vision and hearing tests, psychological and intelligence tests, educational assessments, brain scans, brain wave tests).

Appendix 2: Assessment - Issues For Parents

Previous management and treatment

Who has previously seen your child ? Give details of names, where seen, approximate dates, what treatments were suggested and what happened as a result ? The people involved may include: family doctor, paediatrician, psychologist, private tutor, special education teacher, speech pathologist, optometrist, occupational therapist, physiotherapist.

What have you tried ?

What methods are you currently using to help your child and what have you tried in the past ? Which methods have been useful ? Which strategies have not been effective ?

Details of pregnancy and birth

- Were there any problems in the pregnancy with this child ? Give details.
- What was the nature of the birth ? Were there any complications, and if so, what were these ?
- Was the birth premature or overdue ? What was his birth weight ?
- Were there any problems with him in the first few days or weeks of life? Please give details.

Development

- Did you have concerns about his development or progress ? Give details.
- Indicate any concerns you had in terms of when he:
    - Smiled at you
    - Stood unsupported
    - Said first words
    - Ran steadily
    - Rode a bicycle
    - Tied shoelaces
    - Sat alone
    - Walked alone
    - Talked in sentences
    - Rode a tricycle
    - Dressed himself
    - Learned colours

Medical history

- Give details of any important illnesses which have affected him.
- Indicate the nature of the condition or disability and its treatment.

Appendix 2: Assessment - Issues For Parents

His temperament when he was a younger child

Some children were 'easy to get on with' babies and toddlers whereas others were more 'difficult'. Did he manifest any of the following aspects of temperament when he was younger, and to what extent ?

- Very active fetus (unborn baby)
- Did not like being cuddled
- Poor sleep habits
- Very active or 'busy' toddler
- Cried a lot
- Very active baby
- Colicky and irritable
- Temper tantrums
- Rocked the cot a lot
- Fussy feeder

His later temperament

- Does he show any of the following aspects of temperament, and to what extent ?
  - impatient
  - demands constant attention
  - difficult to keep him satisfied
  - inflexible and stubborn
  - immature or easily led by others
  - attempts to dominate others
  - low frustration tolerance
  - appetite problems
  - lacks motivation
  - has difficulties organising himself
  - reluctant to accept changes in routine
  - lives in the here and now
  - overreacts to criticism or correction
  - self-centred or selfish
  - wants things to be done his way
  - unwilling to listen to suggestions
  - blames others when things go wrong
  - poor sleep pattern
  - procrastinates or puts off decisions
  - poor self esteem
  - has to be encouraged to do things

Family history

- Are there members of his family who have any medical problem or disability that needs attention ? Give details about the condition and its treatment.
- Have any of the following behaviours been a concern for other members of his family ? Who ?
  - problems in paying attention
  - disorganised
  - difficulty in controlling anger
  - moodiness
  - depression
  - impatience or doing things on impulse
  - being restless or fidgety
  - reading or writing problems
  - poor self-esteem
  - alcohol or drug-related problem

Appendix 2: Assessment - Issues For Parents

General concerns about school

Do you have any concerns about his learning or other school activities ? To what extent are the following issues a problem ?

- untidy schoolwork or homework
- leaves homework to last minute
- has trouble keeping up with others
- poor motivation with schoolwork
- lacks confidence with schoolwork
- gets into trouble at school
- dislikes school
- does not complete schoolwork
- not doing as well as he could
- disorganised
- avoids academic work
- gives up easily
- not popular with other students

Specific matters about school

To what extent are you concerned about your child in these specific areas ?

- paying attention
- following instructions
- recalling information
- reading
- spelling
- writing
- mathematics
- drawing and eye-hand coordination
- muscle coordination eg in playing sport or in physical education

- Has he ever been suspended or expelled from school ? Give details.
- Has he received special education or additional help for his schoolwork ? Give details.

Behaviour Questionnaire No.1

To what extent are the following behaviours a problem for him ?

- restless and on the go
- interrupts or disturbs others
- distracted easily
- forgetful
- fiddles with things or fidgets
- moodiness
- acts before thinking - impulsive
- difficulty in paying attention
- poor ability to focus on some activities
- poor ability to complete tasks
- easily frustrated with little things
- unpredictable behaviour

Appendix 2: Assessment - Issues For Parents

Situations

To what extent are the following situations a problem for him in terms of his behaviour and in paying attention ?
- when he plays on his own
- with his mother
- with his father
- when instructions are repeated
- in new or unfamiliar situations
- when he receives one-to-one attention
- when few demands are made on him
- in structured situations
- in stimulating and colourful situations
- when he receives immediate rewards, feedback or consequences
- when watching television or playing with computer games
- familiar situations such as home or school
- when many demands are imposed on him
- when parents are on the telephone
- in public places such as supermarkets
- when playing with several other children or in group situations
- in situations which are boring for him
- situations in which he is not rewarded for effort
- when carrying out tasks which require sustained attention
- activities which demand him to make plans and organise himself

Behaviour Questionnaire No. 2 (Associated Conditions)

To what extent are the following issues a problem ? Give details.
- speech and articulation
- language
- reading
- spelling
- arithmetic or mathematics
- writing
- muscle coordination

- bladder problems
- bowel problems

- jerky or 'twitchy' movements of any part of his body
- unusual utterances, noises or mannerisms involving his voice

Appendix 2: Assessment - Issues For Parents

Behaviour Questionnaire No. 3 (Oppositional and Aggressive Behaviour)

To what extent are these behaviours a concern ?
- loss of temper
- defiant and annoying behaviour
- spiteful behaviour
- deliberate lying and stealing
- truanting from school
- frequent arguing
- angry and resentful
- uses obscene language
- fire setting
- cruelty to animals or people

Other information

Is there any other relevant information which could be helpful ? Give details.

What would you like to see happen ?

What type of help are you seeking and how do you think we can be of help ?

Any questions ?

What questions you would like to have answered ?

Appendix 3 : Assessment - Teacher Issues

APPENDIX 3

ASSESSMENT - TEACHER ISSUES

The teacher's input is vital in the assessment of this student. Your help is greatly appreciated and acknowledged.

Student's name .... Grade ....
School ....

General issues
- Has he ever repeated a grade ? Give details.
- Number of students in the class ....
- Give details about the classroom structure and seating arrangements.

Concerns about his learning and behaviour

What concerns, if any, do you have about his academic performance, achievement, classroom and yard behaviour, self esteem, social adjustment and interaction with other students ?

Is he receiving additional help for any learning, behaviour or related problems ? Please elaborate.

What psychological or educational assessments, if any, have been carried out in the past ? Please elaborate on the findings and summarise the recommendations made. What special programs have been introduced ?

What are his strengths, assets and abilities ?

Comment on his motivation, attitude to work, and any specific difficulties he experiences with academic and non-academic subjects.

Appendix 3 : Assessment - Teacher Issues

Behaviour Questionnaire No.1
To what extent are the following behaviours a problem for him ?
- restless and on the go
- interrupts or disturbs others
- distracted easily
- forgetful
- fiddles with things or fidgets
- moodiness
- trouble in keeping friends
- acts before thinking - impulsive
- difficulty in paying attention
- poor ability to focus on any one activity
- poor ability to complete tasks
- easily frustrated over little things
- unpredictable behaviour

Behaviour Questionnaire No. 2
To what extent do these occur ?
- switches from one activity to another
- other students dislike him
- disturbs activities of other students
- unresponsive to discipline
- has trouble conforming to class rules and routines
- can't wait his turn in games
- acts the clown
- demands a lot of attention

Behaviour Questionnaire No. 3 (Attention and Related Issues)
To what extent are the following matters a problem ?
- avoids doing schoolwork
- needs a lot of supervision
- has difficulty in getting organised
- finds difficulty in planning his work
- doesn't finish things he starts
- procrastinates - puts things off
- lacks motivation to do things
- work habits are sloppy or untidy
- has problems following directions
- works below his true potential
- forgets newly learned information quickly
- repetitive errors in reading, writing, spelling and maths
- difficulty in persisting with certain tasks

Appendix 3 : Assessment - Teacher Issues

- has trouble conforming with class rules and routines
- projects and assignments are incomplete
- has problems keeping up with the rest of the class
- schoolwork not handed in on time
- lacks satisfaction and pride in his schoolwork
- makes excuses for poor quality of work

Situations, tasks and activities

He may have more difficulties in controlling his behaviour or paying attention in certain situations or with particular tasks. Please indicate if any of the following situations create problems in terms of his behaviour or attention. To what extent are these a problem for him ?

- before entering the classroom in the morning
- while carrying out individual desk work
- small group activities
- large group activities eg team games or sports
- during formal didactic teaching or lectures
- during less formal activities such as drama or physical activities
- at recess or lunch in the playground
- during excursions
- during 'quiet time'
- class discussions
- in the mornings
- in the afternoons
- when particular subjects are being taught. Which ones create difficulties ?

Skills and Abilities Checklist

To what extent are you concerned about the following academic skills ?

- Reading comprehension
- Vocabulary
- Word recognition
- Oral expression
- Handwriting - maturity, speed, legibility and neatness

Appendix 3 : Assessment - Teacher Issues

- Handwriting - correct use of punctuation
- Handwriting - correct use of grammar
- Spelling
- Oral comprehension
- Mathematics - understands basic facts and concepts eg addition
- Written calculations
- Copying words and numbers correctly
- General knowledge
- Listening skills

Motor Coordination Skills Checklist

To what extent are you concerned about the following skills ?
- Running, jumping, hopping or skipping
- Pencil control - drawing, colouring in, tracing, printing and writing legibly
- Throwing, catching and batting activities

Speech and Language

To what extent are you concerned about him in the following areas ?
- Extent of vocabulary
- Comprehension
- Pronunciation
- Communication with others
- Fluency of speech

Study Skills

To what extent are you satisfied with the following study skills and habits ?
- Well organised
- Plans what needs to be done and sets priorities
- Identifies the most relevant and important information
- Has a good idea of what the teacher considers is important

Appendix 4 : Benefits Of Medication

APPENDIX 4

BENEFITS OF MEDICATION

The following tables summarise the potential positive effects of medication used in the management of ADD.

Table 1
Medication Improves These Aspects of ADD :

- Ability to focus attention
- Ability to recall information
- Completion of tasks
- Compliance and cooperation
- Fine motor coordination
- Self-control of behaviour
- Self-correcting behaviour
- Alertness
- Ability to control motor activity
- Relevant on-track conversation
- Ability to sustain attention over time
- Ability to persist and stay on task
- Accuracy in carrying out tasks
- Calmness, confidence and relaxation
- Gross motor coordination
- Organisational skills
- Work habits
- Self-esteem and contentment
- Mood

Table 2
Medication Reduces These Aspects Of ADD :

- Impulsive behaviour
- Restlessness and fidgeting
- Errors with academic tasks
- Mental fatigue
- Mood swings
- Immature behaviour
- Defiance and disobedience
- Frustration
- Aggression
- Oppositional behaviour
- Name calling
- Motor activity level
- Daydreaming
- Lying and stealing

Appendix 4 : Benefits Of Medication

As a result of these positive changes there are improvements in the way the parents, brothers and sisters, peers, friends and teachers perceive and view him. These are the secondary positive effects of the medication.

Table 3
Secondary Effects Of Medication

- Other people relate to him in more positive ways
- More popular with other children
- Fewer negative reactions from parents
- Fewer put-downs from others
- Less need to discipline him
- Fewer behaviour problems at school; fewer detentions and suspensions
- Improved cooperation between family members
- Less conflict and stress at home and in the classroom
- Improved school performance
- Improved handwriting and fewer mistakes in written work
- More favourable school reports
- Less disruptive and aggressive behaviour
- Parents and teachers become less defensive or frightened of him

APPENDIX 5

SOME SPECIFIC PSYCHOLOGICAL STRATEGIES

This appendix describes some important practical issues involved in the management of unacceptable behaviour in children. The program is aimed at children whose mental age is between two and ten years. The program must not be used in isolation, and it should preferably be used in conjunction with other treatments such as medication.

This program needs to be carried out properly in order to be effective. It is likely to consume time, energy and effort on the part of the parents. The child's teacher needs to be aware of the program so that similar strategies may be applied at school, and this is likely to encourage a cooperative and consistent approach between home and school.

Summary Of A Behaviour Change Program

A practical behaviour management program will now be presented. A summary of the steps will be given first and this will be followed by details of each of the specific steps.

1 Actively look for signs of acceptable behaviours and work out ways of rewarding them.

2 Determine some basic house rules and know how to give instructions.

3 Work out which specific behaviours need changing.
   Determine when these behaviours are likely to occur.

4 Determine how you will deal with these troublesome behaviours when they occur - the 'time out' procedure.

Appendix 5 : Some Specific Psychological Strategies

1. Actively look for signs of acceptable behaviour

When his acceptable behaviours are rewarded, he is more likely to repeat them. He needs to be rewarded immediately and each time he carries out these positive behaviours. Note that the words 'acceptable' and 'positive' are used, rather than 'angelic', 'fantastic', 'outstanding' or 'extraordinary'.

Unfortunately, some parents reward only excellent behaviour. Some parents find it uncomfortable to give compliments or other rewards. They may not realise the importance of such praise. Other parents go overboard with their praise.

Many parents concentrate only on his negative behaviours and punish their child when he engages in these. All children, even those whose behaviour is intolerable at times, have islands of good behaviour. As pointed out previously, positive behaviour tends to occur in various situations, and parents need to pay special attention to him in these settings.

His positive behaviours must not be taken for granted. Some parents find it difficult to notice his acceptable behaviours and even if they do witness it, they do not reward him because they feel that they should be carried out automatically and without praise. What these parents are actually doing is reinforcing his negative behaviours by providing him with attention during the bad times, and so make it less likely that the positive behaviour will occur again in the future. Research has shown that parents who concentrate only on the negative behaviours see little, if any, improvement in their child's overall behaviour.

The first goal is to increase the occurrence of positive behaviours before considering how to manage more troublesome behaviours. Some parents find it useful to write down specific behaviours and make a special point of rewarding their child when these occur. They actively look and search for positive behaviours and reward him each and every time he engages in them.

Some of the ways of rewarding acceptable behaviours include: *social rewards* including hugs, pats on the back, kiss, clapping, thumbs up, winking, saying 'thank you for ....', 'I like it when you ....'; and *tangible rewards and privileges*

Appendix 5 : Some Specific Psychological Strategies

such as allowing him to play with his favourite toys, tokens eg pocket money, comics, television time, games, reading to him, having a friend sleep over, going out for a meal, and staying up late.

2. Determine some basic house rules and how to give instructions

We all need some rules so that we know what to expect from ourselves and from others. Rules help prevent anarchy and allow us to get on with each other. As pointed out previously, children with ADD are more likely to experience difficulties in responding to rules, requests and instructions.

Because of this, requests and instructions need to be given in a special way. Rules may need to be developed for the daily chores and activities he is expected to carry out. If these are performed properly, he may become better organised.

Some common rules may involve: waking in the morning; bathing; dressing; eating his meals; playing with other children; watching television; visiting other people; doing chores around the home; shopping; homework and studying; brushing his teeth; and going to bed.

Here are some of the important issues involved in giving instructions:

- Get him into a situation in which there are no distractions
- Gain his attention and make direct eye contact with him
- Say clearly what you want him to do and mean what you say
- Act immediately and encourage him to comply with the instruction and supervise him while he is doing it
- Do not accept excuses for not carrying out the request. Remind him that the instruction has to be carried out immediately and stick to your guns. Don't let him wear you down when he uses delay, guilt or other tactics
- Reward him for carrying out the instruction.

3. Work out which specific behaviours need changing

By encouraging his positive behaviours and rewarding him for performing them, some of the more difficult behaviours may decrease in frequency and intensity.

Appendix 5 : Some Specific Psychological Strategies

As pointed out, many parents use negative or punitive methods in an attempt to control his unacceptable behaviours. These strategies often fail and they need to be avoided because they can result in poor self-esteem and are likely to produce more of the negative behaviours in the future.

Some of the methods that are unlikely to be of benefit include negative verbal statements and put-downs such as 'why don't you grow up', 'you're a selfish brat', 'you're hopeless', 'can't you do anything properly', 'why aren't you like your sister .... she always does as she is told'.

Shouting and yelling abusive comments or physical actions such as spanking and hitting, pushing, raising the fist and using other threatening gestures are also unlikely to be of value.

All behaviour occurs in the context of a situation. As already pointed out, children with ADD experience more difficulties in some situations than in others. Careful planning is vital in preventing some of these behaviours from happening in the first place.

Before he enters a particular situation or activity, it is vital that he be given an explanation of the behaviour expected of him. If, for instance, you have to take him shopping or visiting, tell him in specific terms what you expect of him, how he will be rewarded, and what will happen if he doesn't comply. The same needs to be done when it comes to doing homework, chores and when you are on the telephone. The instructions may need to be repeated, sometimes several times, as the situation approaches.

Some irritating behaviours may be ignored if the parents consider them to be minor infringements. Ignoring, however, is sometimes easier said than done.

4. Determine how to deal with the troublesome behaviours when they occur - the 'time out' procedure

'Time out' is a very useful procedure in managing unacceptable behaviours. It basically means taking him away from the situation which triggers or rewards his

Appendix 5 : Some Specific Psychological Strategies

undesirable behaviour, and it also places him in a situation which does not reward him. It allows him to contemplate his actions and also gives the parents an opportunity to cool down and recharge their own batteries.

Step 1 Identify the specific behaviours for which you intend to use time out

Parents need to target the exact behaviours they want to work on. 'Being naughty', 'selfish', 'disruptive' or 'a bad boy' are too general, and such terms may be confusing to him. On the other hand, remarks such as 'pulling your sister's hair', 'throwing the toy car at Rebecca' or 'kicking a hole in the door' are specific behaviours which cannot create confusion for him. Write out a list of the behaviours you wish to modify.

It is best to identify up to three specific negative behaviours only. Quite often other problem areas improve when the identified target behaviours come under his control.

Step 2 Continue using rewards for positive behaviours

Step 3 Decide on the location for time out or where it will take place

Choose some place in which there are no reinforcements. Avoid settings in which there are enjoyable things for him to do. The place should be free of toys, games, books, television, radio and other people. His own room is not a good place because of the positive distractions available to him. The bathroom, toilet or laundry are dull and non-reinforcing places and are often used. Some parents prefer the use of a time out chair facing the corner of a room; this can be useful because his parents can supervise him more closely.

Step 4 Decide on the length of time for the time out

As a general rule, allow one minute of time out for every year of the child's age. Therefore, if he is 7 years old, he would need approximately 7 minutes of time out. It is important not to overstep this time limit.

Appendix 5 : Some Specific Psychological Strategies

Step 5   Explain the new rules to him

Both parents need to sit down with him in a quiet place and at a time when there are no distractions. They must explain the new rules and their new expectations of him in specific terms. This includes details about rewards for acceptable behaviour and time out for unacceptable behaviour.

They may need to explain this several times. It is useful to have the new rules written down in terms that he can understand and for this to be displayed in a prominent place, such as the front of the refrigerator, so that he may be reminded of them.

Step 6   Make sure he really understands the new rules

Time must be taken to ensure that he truly understands the rules. Several explanations may need to be given. It is useful to clarify any issues he may not understand, and for him to reiterate your expectations to ensure that everyone is very clear about what needs to be done.

Step 7   Both parents must carry out the time out procedure

Both parents need to be involved as a team and so reduce the possibility of the use of 'divide and conquer' tactics.

Step 8   Instructing and enforcing him to go to time out when he contravenes the rules

First of all, ask him to stop the undesirable behaviour. Then notice what he does. If he does stop, then reinforce or reward him for listening. If he continues the behaviour, walk up to him, get his attention and give him the warning 'if you don't do as I say, you will be sent to time out'. If he stops, reward him for listening to you. If, on the other hand, he continues the behaviour, make eye contact and, in a firm voice, order him to go to time out immediately.

The instruction to go to time out must be done in a controlled, unemotional, matter-of-fact and firm way.

Appendix 5 : Some Specific Psychological Strategies

Avoid nagging, name calling, asking for explanations, lecturing, shouting and physical methods. (These may actually reinforce his undesirable behaviour because these provide him with attention).

Not all children cooperate with the time out procedure. He may test his parents by using a number of tactics, for example: arguing; promising never to do it again; blaming someone else for his misbehaviour; or denying that he did anything wrong in the first place. These excuses and promises are a ploy to try to get out of time out, and they must be ignored. The parent has an obligation to follow through - no matter what. Otherwise he may continue this type of manipulation, and so make it more difficult to enforce time out in the future.

Some children become quite aggressive and may physically resist time out. The parent may need to use physical means and take him by the wrist or actually carry him to his time out venue. If he is too large and physical force is out of the question, the parent may have to remove additional privileges until he agrees to do his time.

Once placed in time out, other problems may arise. He may throw a tantrum, yell, scream, swear or threaten to leave time out before he is supposed to. The parent must firmly remind him that time out will not start until he stops 'carrying on'. The time out procedure is not started until he is sitting quietly.

If he leaves time out prematurely, the parent should warn him that unless he returns, then he will receive a smack on the bottom. If he does so, then the parent carries out the threat by giving one spank on the bottom. If parents are uncomfortable in doing this, they may remove additional privileges until the required time out is fully served.

He needs to stay in time out for the entire length of time. There must not be any time off for good behaviour and he must not be interrupted during the procedure. After the completion of the time out, he must be instructed to carry out the original instruction. The other parent, if at home, must back up these efforts for time out.

Time out should be carried out each and every time he misbehaves and after a warning is given.

Appendix 5 : Some Specific Psychological Strategies

Time out must be carried out properly to be effective. It may take some time before there is a general improvement in his behaviour. His behaviour may even worsen when the time out procedure is first introduced because he is likely to test out his parents. It may take some time for him to realise that they are committed to this technique.

Some of the mistakes parents make in using the time out procedure include:
- not acting soon enough after the undesirable behaviour occurs, warning him too often or begging him to stop misbehaving
- allowing him to talk his way out of time out
- talking too much or scolding him while placing him in time out
- allowing him to intimidate them into letting him off the hook
- not using rewards for acceptable behaviour. In other words they use time out as the only technique for managing his behaviour

Behaviour change may take several days to weeks because past troublesome behaviour has 'accumulated' over a long time. Old habits die hard, and they may take some time to change.

Consequences for both positive and undesirable behaviours have to be carried out immediately. Parents must not be discouraged and must not give in when they apply time out.

Step 9 Be consistent

He needs a consistent and predictable approach in all areas. He may become confused if he is punished for a misdemeanour on one occasion and is let off the hook at another time for the same behaviour. This may lead to an escalation of his negative behaviour because he learns that he can get away with it at least some of the time, and he is more likely to push things to the limit to test his parents in the hope that they will give in.

Step 10 Determine progress

This means keeping track of the target problem behaviours as well as the positive behaviours. The best way of doing this is to keep an accurate record

Appendix 5 : Some Specific Psychological Strategies

of the number of times each of these occur on a daily basis. This record will enable the parents to determine if their efforts are being effective.

For instance, the effectiveness of time out is based on a reduction of negative behaviours over a period of time. If there is no reduction in these behaviours, then parents should review the way they are carrying out the time out method. They should ask themselves 'are we doing this correctly or are we falling into some of the mistakes in carrying out this procedure ?'

If they consider that they are carrying out the procedure properly, then they may need to try some other method in addition to what they are already doing. If they have any doubts about the procedure, the parents may seek advice from a psychologist who specialises in the area of behaviour management.

If the time out method is working well, then it should be continued.

Appendix 6 : Skills Development

APPENDIX 6

SKILLS DEVELOPMENT

The child with ADD may benefit from specific programs which focus on the development of particular skills. He may not have previously acquired such skills because of the difficulties experienced in controlling his behaviour and paying attention.

These 'new' skills are best learned while his ADD is being treated, say with medication, and while he is better able to focus and sustain his attention. This will allow him to take full advantage of skills development programs. The types of skills which need to be learned depend on the individual requirements of each child. They are best learned and practised in the context of a structured program which is supervised by an appropriate specialist in the field and someone who also understands children with ADD. It is vital that skills also be practised in the child's natural environment, including home and school.

Some of the important skills and their elements are listed below.

Learning Specific Skills

- Pinpointing desired goals
- Determining priorities, making decisions and carrying out plans aimed at working toward these goals
- Identifying the skills required, and the resources and materials needed to reach these goals
- Determining the skills needed to overcome any obstacles to your plans
- Practising the skills regularly
- Rewarding yourself at each step along the way to reaching your goals
- Modifying the physical and social environments so that your efforts are more likely to succeed
- Evaluating your progress regularly and making modifications as necessary
- Asking for, and accepting, positive feedback from others during the process

Appendix 6 : Skills Development

Problem Solving

- Defining the problem
- Exploring alternative solutions
- Setting priorities
- Reviewing alternatives objectively
- Making a decision
- Following through on the decision
- Evaluating the results and other consequences
- Evaluating the strategies used and determining what else needs to be done
- Congratulating and rewarding yourself

Time Management

- Determining main areas of time allotment
- Defining goals clearly
- Setting priorities
- Careful planning
- Preventing and avoiding crises
- Avoiding over commitment
- Avoiding haste by getting it right first time
- Avoiding interruptions
- Avoiding trivial tasks
- Managing indecision and procrastination

Improving Self-Esteem

- Deciding to make a positive change
- Learning positive self-talk and how to compliment yourself
- Ignoring negative messages and thoughts from yourself and others
- Listening actively for positive comments from others
- Making specific positive changes to your behaviour
- Making contact with positive people whom you can trust
- Learning stress management skills

Appendix 6 : Skills Development

Stress Management

There are many different skills which may be learned to help prevent the effects of stress and to manage it when it is inevitable. It is vital that those skills which suit the needs of the individual be identified, practised and applied in real life situations. Some useful stress management skills include:

- Adequate rest
- Avoidance of harmful substances
- Healthy nutrition
- Relaxation skills eg meditation
- Positive self-talk
- Rehearsal
- Rational thinking
- Attitude change
- Communication skills
- Resolving conflict
- Recreation and hobbies
- Regular exercise
- Environmental control
- Personal planning
- Seeking relevant information
- Thought stopping and switching
- Visualisation
- Handling criticism from others
- Making friends
- Making commitments

Control Of Anger And Other Feelings

Getting in touch with your feelings
- Accepting your own emotions
- Learning to accept that you can cope with strong emotions
- Expressing your feelings constructively

Handling Anger
- Accepting that it is okay to feel angry
- Learning positive and more acceptable ways of expressing anger, for example: 'letting it out' in the presence of a trusted friend and explain why you need to 'get it out'; physical activity; screaming; crying; humour; relaxation; avoid stewing over the cause of your anger; avoid those people who may provoke or trigger your anger

APPENDIX 7

VARYING LEARNING STRATEGIES

The child with ADD experiences a number of difficulties with self-motivation, selective and sustained attention, initiation and persistence of effort, and completion of certain tasks. These disabilities can greatly affect his learning and academic performance. He is also likely to become quickly satiated or accustomed to presentations, activities, rewards and feedback if they are repeated in a monotonous and unchanging way.

One of the teacher's main tasks is to try to assist the child overcome these difficulties. Teachers can greatly influence him in very positive ways by modifying the learning environment (see Chapter 14: 'Educational Strategies'), and by varying and modifying the ways in which they involve children in learning experiences. They may also modify the types of materials used and the group structure of the class.

Such variations in methods of learning strategies are likely to improve his motivation, enhance his ability to attend to tasks, enable him to complete his work and improve his performance. The strategies listed below need to be rotated or changed frequently to prevent the potential problems of satiation and habituation. The same strategies also work very well for children who do not have ADD. But they are vital for the child with ADD.

Teachers may need to assess their current methods of providing positive learning experiences for their students. They may consider making necessary modifications to their teaching styles and methods, and introduce strategies which are more suitable for the child with ADD and which will also benefit other students.

The following lists suggests a variety of approaches which should be of benefit to the child with ADD. They will enable him to take increasing control over a number of his difficulties.

Appendix 7 : Varying Learning Strategies

Type Of Procedure

Teacher directed
- Lecture or didactic teaching
- Use of stimulus materials
- Student talks
- Mini lecture
- Handouts
- Worksheets or questionnaires

Demonstration
- Displaying a specific technique
- Rehearsing
- Coaching

Group learning
- Skills practice
- Discussion
- Buzz groups
- Learning groups
- Brainstorming issues and solutions
- Student panels
- Specific task groups
- Question and answer sessions

Individual learning
- Background reading
- Research
- Negotiating work contracts
- Interviews and surveys
- Learning centres
- Homework

Structured experiences
- Role playing
- Case study
- Exercises
- Excursions and field studies
- Making models and displays
- Drama
- Critical incident
- Games
- Social skills games
- Making tapes or videos

Group Structure

- Whole group
- Circle
- Fish bowl
- Small group
- Horseshoe
- Self-select groups
- Pairs
- Rows
- Trios or quartets
- Table group

Appendix 7 : Varying Learning Strategies

Materials And Resources

- Chalk and board
- Pamphlets
- Overhead transparencies
- Television programs
- Radio programs
- Butcher's paper
- Books and booklets
- Projector and slides
- Video programs
- Audio cassette

REFERENCES

American Psychiatric Association (1991): *DSM-IV Options Book: Work In Progress. Task Force On DSM-IV.* Washington, DC, American Psychiatric Association.

Barkley, R.A. (1987). *Defiant Children: A Clinician's Manual for Parent Training.* New York: Guildford Press.

Barkley, R.A. (1990). *Attention Deficit Hyperactivity Disorder: A Clinical Handbook for Diagnosis and Treatment.* New York: Guildford Press.

Barkley, R.A. (1991). *Attention Deficit Hyperactivity Disorder: A Clinical Workbook.* New York: Guildford Press.

Children with Attention Deficit Disorders (1991). *Attention Deficit Disorders : Understanding Through Education. Proceedings from the Third Annual Ch.A.D.D. Conference on Attention Deficit Disorders for Parents, Educators, and Health-Care Professionals. Held on September 19-20, 1991 in Washington, DC.* Plantation, Florida: Children with Attention Deficit Disorders.

Levine, E.D., Carey, W.B., Crocker, A.C., & Gross, R.T. (1983). *Developmental - Behavioral Pediatrics.* Philadelphia: W.B. Saunders.

Nash, H. (1994). *Medication for Attention Deficit Disorder.* Unpublished Manuscript.

Nash, H. (1993). *Tourette Syndrome.* Unpublished Manuscript.

Parker, H. (1989). *The ADD Hyperactivity Workbook for Parents, Teachers and Kids.* Plantation, Florida: Impact Publications.

Parker, H. (1992). *The ADD Hyperactivity Handbook for Schools.* Plantation, Florida: Impact Publications.

Serfontein, G. (1990). *The Hidden Handicap.* Australia: Simon & Schuster.

Serfontein, G. (1994). *ADD in Adults.* Australia: Simon & Schuster.

Wender, P.H. (1987). *The Hyperactive Child, Adolescent, and Adult: Attention Deficit Disorder Through the Life Span.* New York: Oxford University Press.

Zametkin, A.J., Nordahl, T.E., Gross, M., King, A.C., Semple, W.E., Rumsey, J., Hamburger, S., & Cohen, R.M. (1990). Cerebral Glucose Metabolism in adults with Hyperactivity of childhood onset. *New England Journal of Medicine, 323,* 1361-1366.